Alzheimer's Disease

The Dignity Within

A Handbook for Caregivers, Family, and Friends

Alzheimer's Disease

The Dignity Within

A Handbook for Caregivers, Family, and Friends

Patricia R. Callone, MA, MRE
Barbara C. Vasiloff, MA
Connie Kudlacek, BS
Janaan Manternach, D MIN
Roger A. Brumback, MD

Demos Medical Publishing, LLC
386 Park Avenue South
New York, New York 10016

Visit our website at
www.demosmedpub.com

Design and production: Reyman Studio
Copyeditor: Joann Woy
Indexing: Joann Woy
Printer: Capital City Press

Memories in the Making is a copyrighted product of the
Alzheimer's Association of Orange County, New Jersey.

Made in the United States of America
Library of Congress Cataloging-in-Publication Data

Alzheimer's disease : the dignity within : a handbook for caregivers,
family, and friends / Patricia R. Callone ... [et al.].
p. cm.
Includes index.
ISBN 1-932603-13-1 (alk. paper)
1. Alzheimer's disease—Patients—Care—Handbooks, manuals, etc.
2. Alzheimer's disease—Patients—Family relationships—Handbooks, manuals, etc.
3. Caregivers–Handbooks, manuals, etc. I. Callone, Patricia R.
RC523.A397598 2005362.196'831–dc22
                        2005009593

We dedicate this handbook to the
thousands of caregivers, family members, and friends
of persons with Alzheimer's disease or related
dementia everywhere. May this handbook be a resource for
them as they care for their loved ones.

Caregiving

"A spiritual practice as one human being dares to enter into relationship and service for the benefit of another."
— Mary Pauluk, Chaplain
St. John Lutheran Home, Springfield, Minnesota

Not many of us have been trained to be caregivers. Yet, in a way, we all become caregivers at sometime in our lives. Caregiving is a normal part of life. There is no absolute right or wrong way of doing it. Each caregiver and each family develops special relationships and caregiving practices that help them succeed.

In her book, *And Thou Shalt Honor: The Caregiver's Companion*, Beth Witrogen McLeod says, "We've been called to tend to others, not to martyr ourselves in the process." She goes on to say, "This [caregiving] can be a precious time if we approach the caregiving role as a calling rather than as an obstacle to achieving personal goals. Caregiving is truly a spiritual practice, a nonlinear path with heart. We are asked to expand ourselves and be open to change. We are asked to comfort, to guide, to love. We are asked to listen, to reassure, to advocate. Most of all, we are asked to trust life in a way we never thought possible. What makes caregiving appear difficult is the inner journey, the one that requires us to summon the courage and flexibility to relate to life in an unfamiliar but more expansive way. This is new territory for most of us; it shows us where we have closed down to what life has to offer, and how much work is necessary to care for ourselves while caring for others...."

Preface

This handbook is a reference guide for caregivers, family members, and friends of people affected by Alzheimer's disease or related dementia. For many years, the literature concerning Alzheimer's disease has concentrated on the physical and mental losses that occur as the disease progresses.

The world is still looking for a cure or for ways to halt the harm done to the brain by the disease, but today more hope exists for those seeking drug therapies during the various stages. Researchers and scientists around the world are looking for ways to cure, defer, or halt the progression of the disease.

More emphasis is being placed on how each of us can maintain the health of our brains through healthy lifestyles, including diet, exercise, and attention to our environment. There have been—and there will be more—advances in understanding and finding cures for this disease as additional financial resources are dedicated to research worldwide.

The nonphysical world—the inner world of the person affected by Alzheimer's disease—is being given more attention by such scholars as Dr. Steven R. Sabat, author of *The Experience of Alzheimer's Disease: Life through a Tangled Veil* and Professor of Psychology at Georgetown

University. Dr. Sabat and others, such as Dr. Stephen Post, author of *The Moral Challenges of Alzheimer's*, are concentrating on how the disease affects an individual's "personal identity" and "sense of self." Researchers, scientists, and psychologists are bringing to us all new insights about the inner world of those affected by the disease.

It is a hopeful time for those who believe that the "essence within" the person with Alzheimer's disease can be touched and empowered throughout the different stages of the disease. If caregivers, family members, and friends concentrate more on this "essence within" or the "dignity within," then the task of caregiving, though rigorous, can be lightened. Caregivers, family members, and friends can enjoy the skills, talents, joys, and humor that remain intact throughout the progression of the disease.

The five authors of this handbook care deeply about people affected by Alzheimer's disease or related dementia and their caregivers. Our perspective focuses on the mental and physical functions that remain in spite of those losses that can never be recovered. We believe both caregivers and people affected by Alzheimer's disease can live with a sense of dignity, importance, and self-esteem.

We believe that people with Alzheimer's disease and related dementia:

   ♦ Can continue to have meaningful and productive lives through engaging in activities and interests that they have enjoyed and learned throughout their lives, for as long as various functions of the brain remain intact.

   ♦ Should retain their power of choice to say "yes" and "no" as long as possible, for the good of everyone, including those affected by the disease, caregivers, family members, and friends.

We believe caregivers:

   ♦ Will be empowered to do a better job of caregiving if they understand that Alzheimer's disease is truly a disease affecting the different parts of the brain and that people with the disease cannot control some of their behaviors as the disease progresses.

   ♦ Will be more tolerant and patient if they reflect on the "sense of self" that remains in the person affected by the disease.

   ♦ Can make healthy decisions during all stages of the progression of Alzheimer's disease if they will reflect on the three styles of acting as outlined in this handbook.

❧ Need to learn how to take care of themselves and develop meaningful lives during the caregiving process.

The text in this handbook is arranged in five parts. Part I covers the challenges of being a caregiver and offers some solutions; Part II tells the personal story of the relationship between a husband and wife as they cope and come to terms with the husband's Alzheimer's disease; Part III relates true stories of the relationships that develop between persons affected by Alzheimer's disease, their caregivers, family members, and friends; Part IV covers the three most effective caregiving styles; and Part V explores the changes to the brain that occur in Alzheimer's disease.

Our greatest desire is that the time you spend with this handbook will have a positive benefit on the lives of those affected by Alzheimer's disease or related dementia and their caregivers, family members, and friends.

Acknowledgments

THANK YOU Florence Andersen Callone, Clara Callone Gryva, and Manuel Joseph Callone—all of whom have been an inspiration for this handbook.

THANK YOU Joyce Bunger, Maureen Crouchley, Lynn Denzler, Carol Feelhaver, Bill Flynn, Paul Keating, Michele King, Sofia Kock, Gene Kudlacek, Bonnie Lingard, Marie Micheletto, RSM, Ruth Purtilo, PhD, Tia Schoenfeld, Maureen Waldron, Collen Warin, and Carolyn Wright for helping us focus on caregivers' needs and the needs of their families.

THANK YOU Mary Ann Urbashich, Associate Director, Library Projects, Green-Field Library and Resource Center of the Alzheimer's Association, for close editing of parts of the handbook.

THANK YOU Mary Nash and Lynn Schneiderman of the Creighton University Reinert Alumni Memorial Library for assistance with identifying quotations.

THANK YOU Alzheimer's Association, for sharing knowledge and compassion in numerous ways. Because of the Association's work, persons with Alzheimer's disease or related dementia, their caregivers, and family members have hope for new resources in the future.

Contents

Part I. Being a Caregiver: Challenges and Solutions

The Special Journey of Caregivers to Persons with Alzheimer's Disease or Related Dementia

A Dozen Tips for Caregivers

Part III. True Stories: Relationships between Persons Affected by the Disease, Their Caregivers, Family Members, and Friends

About the Illustrations

In 1986, artist, board member and caregiver Selly Jenny, whose
mother had Alzheimer's disease, began to explore the use of an art
program to learn how much dementia patients could reveal about
themselves through the medium of art. Most had never painted
before, yet the response was uniformly positive. A new approach
was implemented, and the Memories in the Making art program was
born. It has grown into a calendar, a manual, an art exhibit, note
cards, and more. It is produced by the Alzheimer's Association of
Orange County and is enjoying international recognition. The paintings reproduced in this book are from Memories in the Making.

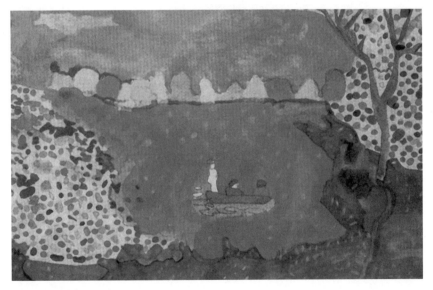

"Spring Fishing" by Joe

Joe lived in the East when he was a child, so this picture could be of Central Park in
New York City, but he is not sure. This "dot" form of painting appears in most
Alzheimer's patients' works. Their paintings have the same look no matter where
they are made. This dot-painting phenomenon is associated with a stage in the
progression of the disease. Sooner or later, "pointillism" becomes the painting
technique of choice in Alzheimer's patients.

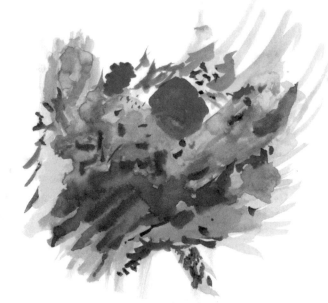

"Flowers" by Peggy

Peggy is a sophisticated woman with intelligent blue eyes. She never had an opportunity to be creative artistically until she participated in the Memories in the Making program. She didn't know she possessed her artistic ability until then. The Memories in the Making creative art program emphasizes how much talent and strength still remain in the human spirit of a person with Alzheimer's disease.

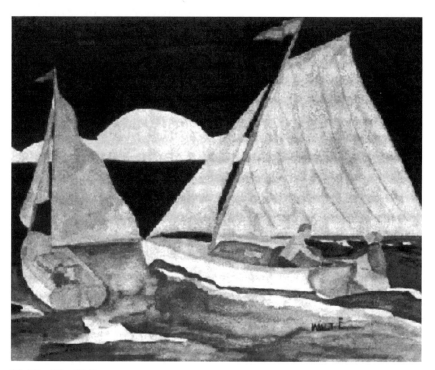

"Sailing" by Walt

Walt had never painted. Now he has become an accomplished artist. Memories are stored deep within us. They return from nowhere, inspired by a scent, a phrase or the sound of a melody. They emerge and take us into another place or time. Our memory bank is always there to help us cope with today's experiences. The Memories art program allows the person to communicate a hidden joy.

Being a Caregiver: Challenges and Solutions

Meet Patricia (Pat) Callone, MA, MRE

In one way or another I have been a caregiver since I was 8 years old. I am an only child who cared for my parents through multiple sclerosis, cancer, and Alzheimer's disease and have been a primary caregiver for Alzheimer's disease to both my mother and father, and a secondary caregiver to my aunt (my cousin was her primary caregiver). My mother died from Alzheimer's disease and related complications in 1990. My aunt died from Alzheimer's disease in 2001. My father is still living and has Alzheimer's disease. He is in the moderate stage of the disease.

Each caregiving situation has been a unique experience. To be a caregiver to someone who is physically ill and to be a caregiver to someone with dementia are two sides of the same coin. In both instances the caregiver is asked to serve, but in different ways. It seems to me that one of the most important tasks confronting a caregiver is to find information about the disease and how it affects the person physically and mentally. When caregivers, family members, and friends have accurate information, they can be the best possible caregivers.

Over the years I have become a wiser companion to others in their caregiving journeys, but only if I learned new ways to be a better caregiver myself. Reading, research, and my personal experience have led me to draw conclusions about certain aspects of being a caregiver to persons with Alzheimer's disease or related dementia.

Additionally a new interest—dare I say even a passion—is developing: finding and nurturing "the dignity within" persons affected by the disease. This single tenet has been the driving force behind my caregiving experiences and the eventual decision to prepare this handbook.

During my eighteen years' experience with this disease, I have read a great deal about long goodbyes. Most of the information concerns behavior management and the impact the disease has on the family. There was very little about the self-awareness or preserved abilities and skills of persons with Alzheimer's disease that satisfied my curiosity or clearly spoke to the concept of the "dignity within."

To me the "dignity within" means finding and nurturing the remaining functions, abilities, gifts, and skills of persons who have Alzheimer's disease throughout the progression of the disease: through the early-to-mild, the moderate, and the severe stages.

For six years I have served on the Board of Directors of the Alzheimer's Association Midlands Chapter and have been greatly enriched and supported by the staff as well as had opportunities to attend national and international conferences. Without the support of this organization I would never have made it through some of the most difficult times of my caregiving journey.

I am currently Vice President for Institutional Relations at Creighton University in Omaha, Nebraska, and have many opportunities to meet with colleagues, researchers, physicians, faculty, and staff members who are deeply interested in the latest research and care of persons with dementia. They are interested not only because of their professional interests, but also because many are involved as caregivers.

That is why I asked some very talented friends if they would contribute to a handbook for caregivers, family members, and friends of persons with Alzheimer's disease or related dementia. My vision was that we would develop a handbook that would be a resource to do the following:

1. encourage caregivers to take care of themselves;
2. offer caregivers reflections on crucial questions;
3. help caregivers find better ways to communicate with their loved ones;

4. provide caregivers information about the physical dimensions of the disease that could be clearly understood;
5. point out the functions and abilities that can be nourished throughout the progression of the disease.

Taking care of self and nurturing the functions that remain throughout the progression of the disease leads to acknowledging the "dignity within" both caregivers and persons with Alzheimer's disease or related dementia.

I knew Barbara C. Vasiloff, co-founder and President of Discipline With Purpose, Inc.; Connie Kudlacek, Executive Director of the Alzheimer's Association Midlands Chapter; Dr. Roger A. Brumback, Professor of Pathology and Psychiatry and Chairman of the Department of Pathology at the Creighton University School of Medicine; and author and educator, Janaan Manternach. Because of their expertise these friends could easily meet the challenge of developing a handbook I envisioned.

Together we are sharing our insights and experiences, which are much like those of other caregivers and professionals, in this handbook. Through the work of this team, I have learned many remarkable things: from Barbara, new ways to communicate with my father; from Connie, new resources and insights concerning caregivers and persons with the disease; from Roger, new information about how Alzheimer's disease affects the brain; and from Janaan, a companion caregiver, new insights about a couple's relationship while living with Alzheimer's disease.

The Special Journey of Caregivers to Persons with Alzheimer's Disease or Related Dementia

In the United States, Alzheimer's disease is the fourth leading cause of death after heart disease, cancer, and stroke. Because we are living longer due to medical advances, more and more of us will be called upon to be caregivers for someone in our families or our friends who need special care. The medical community is also finding that persons at younger ages can have Alzheimer's disease or related dementia in their 40's, 50's, 60's, and 70's. Statistics tell us that possibly one out of two persons over the age of 85 has dementia. Alzheimer's disease is the most common form of dementia.

PERSONS WITH ALZHEIMER'S DISEASE:

For the person with Alzheimer's disease, the symptoms depend not only on the changes in the brain but also on the overall condition of the person and the environment in which the person affected with dementia lives.

Although there are commonalities, individuals affected with Alzheimer's disease or related dementia experience the disease uniquely. The disease progresses at its own rate and the deterioration does not occur in a lock-step, uniform pattern.

Sometimes it is helpful to divide the progression of the disease into stages so that the disease can be more easily understood. These divisions are like describing the early stages of a child's growth: for example, the "terrible two's" to indicate possible behavior patterns during that stage of development.

"Staging" of the illness serves the purpose of providing guidelines for assessment. "Staging" can be helpful when making a plan for continuous care in order to maximize the person's abilities and dignity. Most of the time the onset of the disease is very subtle. Only in retrospect does the family put the pieces together and recognize when the onset of the disease occurred. Different people divide the progression of Alzheimer's disease into three, four, or five stages. This handbook collapses several of those categorizations into just three stages which we believe are easier to conceptualize: the early-to-mild stage, the moderate stage, and the severe stage.

Persons with Alzheimer's disease do not necessarily move through all stages. Alzheimer's disease is usually only one of a number of physical ailments that individuals experience. There can be other physical complications such as pneumonia, cancer, or heart disease that alter the course of the disease and cause early death.

There are people in the early-to-mild stage of the disease who are willing to talk about their experiences. There are some who are eager to talk about their experiences during the diagnosis of the disease and how they see themselves losing some of their abilities. At the same time, they want us to know what they still can do and how they want to be treated.

At international, regional, and local meetings I have been privileged to hear persons with Alzheimer's disease and their caregivers speak about their experiences with the disease. What persons with Alzheimer's disease want most is to be treated with the dignity they deserve. One woman said, "I have Alzheimer's disease. I've lost my memory, but I haven't lost my mind."

Another person with the disease gave this response: "I want to have a full life. I used to have many responsibilities and be in charge of many tasks. I want to do meaningful work and be useful to others. Don't just give me envelopes to lick and think that I am happy doing that. I can still do some things well."

Evidence of this strong desire to contribute and do meaningful work can be found in the art works throughout this handbook. Each picture was created by a person with Alzheimer's disease who participated in the Memories in the Making© art program of the Alzheimer's Association. Their works are a tribute to the life and dignity that seek to be expressed in persons with Alzheimer's disease.

PERSONS WITH ALZHEIMER'S DISEASE AND THEIR FAMILIES:

Unfortunately, in our society there is a stigma attached to Alzheimer's disease. Many persons diagnosed with the disease and their families do not want to acknowledge they have it because of the stigma society places on them. Perhaps this is true because there are no Alzheimer's disease survivors to talk about how the disease affected them personally and their families.

Family relationships can also be challenging. If relationships are healthy and caring within a family before someone is diagnosed with Alzheimer's disease, the relationships will most likely be healthy and caring during the progression of the disease. If relationships are unhealthy and non-supportive in families before someone has Alzheimer's disease, they probably will be unhealthy and non-supportive during the progression of the disease.

Birth order also plays a role in the caregiving process. An only child generally feels a strong responsibility to take on the role of caregiver since there is no one else to do it. This is especially true of an only girl child. Women are still seen as carrying the responsibilities of being "caregivers" in our society. An only son can feel the responsibility of caring for his parents, but if he is married, the responsibility can easily fall to his wife.

The oldest child can often be expected to assume the responsibilities for parents' care by other siblings. Tension can arise if other family members do not support the decisions made by the oldest child. Middle children are not usually the primary caregivers for parents unless over the years the family dynamics have shifted in that direction. If middle children are closer in distance to the parent needing care, then they can take responsibility and inform other family members about the caregiving process.

Some families call "family forums" to discuss how the care of the person with the disease should be carried out. The person with the disease is often present and should have a say in the overall plans with the family. This gives the person with the disease the dignity he or she deserves. This can be very helpful to the person with the disease and the primary caregiver who acts on behalf of the entire family.

There are general stresses that can impact primary caregivers of persons with Alzheimer's disease or related dementia. An awareness of these stresses can help us know ourselves and understand our inner world and consciousness. Better care for the loved one and ourselves will follow as a result.

Stresses for the Caregiver:

- Caregivers can themselves become exhausted and sick in the process of caring for a loved one.
- Caregivers can sometimes feel trapped and/or "second guess" their decisions.
- Caregivers do not always recognize the signs of the early-to-mild stage of Alzheimer's disease, and these early signs can be just as confusing to caregivers as to persons affected by the disease.
- Caregivers need help to learn not to dwell on the losses that occur in the progression of the disease but instead to concentrate on the functional capabilities that still remain and can be used and enjoyed. Those capabilities are to be cherished, and the person is to be honored and given dignity throughout his/her lifetime.
- Family finances can become depleted and financial support from the government and health insurance industry do not adequately assist the real needs of persons with dementia and their families.
- The medical profession does not always understand the position of caregivers and that sometimes caregivers need as much, or more, attention than persons diagnosed with dementia.

In addition, specific challenges for caregivers arise at the different stages of Alzheimer's disease.

EARLY-TO-MILD STAGE OF ALZHEIMER'S DISEASE

The Early-To-Mild Stage can last for a variable period of time—often from 3 to 5 years.

The person has trouble remembering. The person with early-to-mild dementia can often describe his or her problems clearly. Persons with early-to-mild dementia can continue to do most of the things they have always done. (See Part V. Changes in the Brain.) The Alzheimer's Association has many brochures that more fully explain the progression of the disease.

In the Early-To-Mild Stage of Alzheimer's disease or related dementia, the Caregiver has these awarenesses and concerns:

- The caregiver observes the Loved One and realizes there is a problem. The caregiver is confused about what to do because of the fluctuation between "good" and "bad" days.
- The caregiver wants to know what is wrong and seeks diagnosis so he or she can fix it.
- The caregiver usually assumes more responsibility for the care of the individual and takes over some of the duties of the person with Alzheimer's disease or related dementia.
- The caregiver sometimes feels overwhelmed and embarrassed by the person with the disease and treats the person as if he or she does not understand what is going on. The caregiver can become ashamed, or feel guilty or angry.
- The caregiver can become overprotective and not let the person make choices he or she is capable of making.
- The caregiver can anticipate the loss of a reciprocal relationship with the person who has the disease and recognizes his or her lack of knowledge about long-term plans for personal and health care of the person with dementia.

The Caregiver needs:

- Creative insight to find ways to help the loved one feel productive.
- Personal support from family and friends; too often the family can withdraw from previously supportive relationships because things are not going well.
- Community services and resources from the local Alzheimer's chapter or Office on Aging to discuss what is happening.
- Friends who will bring humor into his or her life.
- Family who will pick up some duties of the caregiver so the caregiver does not become overextended.
- Family and friends who will help the caregiver celebrate life with the person who has the disease as well as with the extended family—engaging in birthday celebrations, weddings, and holiday festivities.

MODERATE STAGE OF ALZHEIMER'S DISEASE

The Moderate Stage can last from 3 to 5 years and the person is one step further in the progression of the disease. (See Part V. Changes in the Brain.) In this stage of the disease the brain deteriorates more and personality changes can occur.

In the Moderate Stage of Alzheimer's disease or related dementia, the Caregiver has these awarenessess and concerns:

- The caregiver becomes more frustrated. Even with the additional care that is being given to the person with dementia, the individual is getting worse.
- The caregiver neglects social and family roles and frequently begins to neglect his or her own health. The caregiver realizes the need to access formal services for the person with dementia and focuses more on the provision of care than on the supervision of care.
- The caregiver becomes more anticipatory of needed care than reactive and seeks help to understand services provided by different assisted living facilities, nursing home facilities, and their costs.
- The caregiver understands the family and the person with Alzheimer's disease need to prepare a plan for long-term personal care and prepare for the costs of the care.
- The family needs to determine who will be given the Durable Power of Attorney for health care and finances. Usually the primary caregiver has these powers, but these powers could be shared with others.

The Caregiver needs:

- To take good care of self—socially, emotionally, and spiritually.
- To have outlets for fun and relaxation.
- To have family and friends distract the caregiver from caregiving responsibilities.
- To get regular physical and dental exams.
- To set aside some time for quiet reflection, prayer and fun.
- To review information on how Alzheimer's disease affects the brain.
- To distinguish fact from feeling as he or she interacts with loved ones.

SEVERE STAGE OF ALZHEIMER'S DISEASE

The duration of the severe stage of the disease depends on the overall condition of the individual. In the severe stage the person becomes relatively non-functional and is often confined to bed. (See Part V. Changes in the Brain.)

In the Severe Stage of Alzheimer's disease or related
dementia the Caregiver has these awarenesses:

- The caregiver focuses on the comfort of the loved one rather than prolongation of life and addresses end-of-life issues such as resuscitation and quality of life.
- The caregiver allows family members and friends to talk and work through their own grief with special attention to honoring the wishes of the loved one with Alzheimer's disease.
- The caregiver feels guilty if the loved one has had to move from the home to an assisted living facility or nursing home.
- The caregiver becomes more frustrated and has feelings of failure if the caregiver has not acquainted himself or herself with the progression of the disease.
- The caregiver anticipates the loss of the loved one with sadness and can become exhausted because of physical caregiving and internal stress.
- The caregiver can feel abandonment or isolation if she or he did not maintain support systems of family, friends, and/or a faith community.

The Caregiver needs:

- Someone to listen to him or her without judging or trying to problem-solve.
- Family, friends, and faith communities to understand the physical, spiritual, and social needs of the caregiver.
- Outlets to laugh and to enjoy parts of life away from caregiving responsibilities.
- Kindness and compassion from friends, family, and medical professionals.
- Family members to support and reinforce difficult decisions that must be made.
- Understanding in the workplace since the caregiver can become distracted at work because of caregiving responsibilities.
- Encouragement to take vacation and sick time as allowed in order to have the energy to sustain the responsibilities of all his or her roles in life.

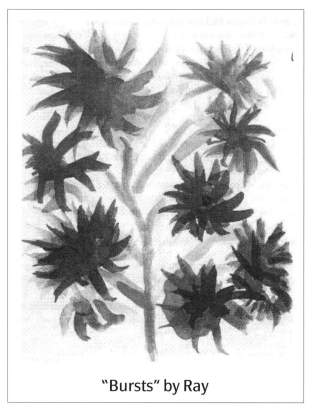

"Bursts" by Ray

Ray experiences loss of verbal communication, but when he is in the Memories in the Making art program and experiencing the support of others in similar situations, his painting gives him a voice. Alzheimer's dementia brings with it a flood of failures and losses. The Memories in the Making art program does not acknowledge failure. Each picture is important and valid.

Through all the stages of Alzheimer's disease, caregivers need to take good care of themselves so they can be the best caregivers possible.

Again, Beth Witrogen McLeod speaking to caregivers: "... Whatever path you choose, please remember this: You are never alone. Every act of kindness counts. Love is always stronger than fear. If you are among those in search of answers to the stresses and confusions inherent in caregiving, I say: 'This **is** your life now. Live it fully in the present. Stay connected to love, which is the heart of caregiving, and your journey will be rewarded many times over.'" (From the Introduction to *And Thou Shalt Honor: The Caregiver's Companion*.)

IN SUMMARY, CAREGIVERS NEED TO TAKE CARE OF THEMSELVES—THEIR MINDS, THEIR BODIES, AND THEIR SPIRITS

Mind—Get the information you need to understand what the disease is doing to the person with dementia. Understand that the person's actions are many times the result of the progression of the disease in the brain. Ask for assistance from friends and professionals.

Body—Eat right, sleep enough, exercise daily, laugh often.

Spirit—Take time to nourish your spirit daily; reflect/pray often during the day; ask for help; continue to take part in your family's activities as often as you can.

With reflection, caregivers can take time to see the whole picture of what they want the caregiving experience to be for themselves, the persons for whom they are caring, their families, and friends.

A Dozen Tips for Caregivers

1. Consider Your Strengths as a Caregiver

A coach once said: "I try to look at the strengths of a player and ask the player to perfect those strengths . . . rather than concentrate on the deficits too much." What are your strengths as a caregiver?

- Do you have a sense of humor?
- Are you patient?
- Can you be quiet with the person?
- Are you a good listener?
- Do you get upset, but then apologize?
- Do you make time for the person with dementia?
- Are you thoughtful? Do you think of surprises for others?
- Have you learned that repeating a phrase or idea over and over again is part of the disease and that the person with dementia does not realize he or she is repeating the same questions or phrases?
- Have you learned enough about Alzheimer's disease to nurture the remaining talents and capabilities of the person?
- What do you bring to the person with dementia that enhances his or her life?

Don't be distracted by your limitations to the extent that you become an ineffective caregiver. Every person has some special strengths. Think about what your strengths are. Capitalize on your strengths and use them to make others and yourself comfortable and happy.

> *Life is like 'A Cup of Tea.'*
> *It's how you make it.*
> —Irish Blessing

2. Consider the Strengths of Others

What is the disposition of the person for whom you are caring? Happy? Cooperative? Interested in you, the family, history, the news?

What intellectual capabilities and senses can be stimulated in the person? Does the person enjoy looking at pictures in family albums? Talking about the past? Visiting the grocery store? Visiting a garden shop? Going to a hardware store? Drawing, listening to music?

In what ways can you take delight in the person with dementia? Don't be distracted by the person's limitations to the extent that you cannot enjoy him/her. Although parts of the brain are affected by the disease, other parts still remain healthy and can function normally. Help stimulate the healthy functions and everyone will be happier.

How can the person feel useful? Create opportunities for him/her to be needed and wanted. Help develop the person's self-esteem whenever possible. Here are two stories that show ways to help persons with Alzheimer's disease or related dementia be happy and healthy.

- One day some women in a nursing home were becoming more and more anxious. A staff member asked one of them if she wanted to help fold some laundry. She did, and others followed. They wanted to do something useful . . . something they were used to doing. The women made a habit of helping fold the laundry and their anxiety decreased. They were physically tired at the end of the day and slept better during the night.
- A gentleman in the severe stage of Alzheimer's disease, who needed help with feeding, could still play the clarinet if held to his lips. The music he produced was almost exactly the same as that he had played in his younger years at the height of his career. What the person has overlearned or done repeatedly during the time he/she was healthier can still be accomplished.

For caregivers, it is important to remember that if we don't like the way things are, we can look for ways to make things different. Even if we cannot change our circumstances, we can change the way we

THINK about them. Our perspectives can shift from emphasizing what persons with Alzheimer's disease cannot do to what they can do.

The man who goes alone can start today; but he who travels
with another must wait until the other is ready.
                                          —Henry David Thoreau

3. Evaluate Your Activities

Consider which relationships and activities are life-giving for you. Consider which relationships are draining for you at this time. Drop those you do not have time for now and keep those that are nurturing. Here are three situations that you might evaluate as you accept more caregiving responsibilities:

- At holiday time (Thanksgiving, the New Year's season, the Fourth of July, etc.) continue the activities that give you most enjoyment and new energy. Drop those that take too much time, are draining, or can be handled by someone else. Maybe it is time for another family member to host the dinner or picnic.
- If you have volunteered in a number of organizations, but now your energy is needed for your caregiving responsibilities, explain to those that call you for assistance that you hope to be able to help the organization at another time, but it is not possible right now.
- If you need quiet time, time to rest, shop, or get groceries, exercise, or just to get away, contact the chapter of the Alzheimer's Association in your area and inquire about respite programs that may be available. Respite can provide assistance to a caregiver so he/she has time away from caregiving responsibilities to take care of himself/herself.

Remember, if you have a reputation for always "being there" for others, you will feel uncomfortable the first time you have "to let go of something" or perhaps say "no" to an activity you have always done. By doing so, however, you are breaking out of your comfort zone to create a new pattern or routine. Remind yourself that when you refocus your life, you can always pick up the activities you dropped because of caregiving responsibilities.

One ought every day at least, to hear a little song,
read a good poem, see a fine picture and if possible,
speak a few reasonable words.
                                          —Goethe

4. *Deal with Hurt*

Many times our feelings can get hurt in the caregiving process. This is especially true when caring for a person with Alzheimer's disease or related dementia. You should remember that Alzheimer's disease affects certain parts of the brain causing not only memory loss but forgetfulness. Often the person is insensitive and demanding; unable to realize the effect his or her behavior has on others.

Here is a situation that exemplifies forgetfulness and insensitivity:

> Janice's father has season tickets for a prestigious college football team. One Friday he calls Janice and offers the tickets to her family. Janice is pleased because her three teenagers will be delighted to go.
>
> On Saturday her father calls and asks, "Where are the football tickets for this afternoon's game?" Janice responds, "You gave them to me yesterday, Dad, and the children are just getting ready to go now." Her father replies, "I didn't give you those tickets. You took them. I want them back . . ."

When something like this happens, try to take a moment and differentiate the facts from the feelings. Say to yourself, "What are the facts here? What am I feeling?"

- The fact is: My father is responding like this because of Alzheimer's disease.
- The feeling is: "I am hurt because he is treating me like this."
- The fact is: "He doesn't remember he gave me the tickets yesterday. He doesn't mean to upset me. His forgetfulness is beginning to cause me and my family problems. I must remember he is acting like this because of the disease."

When you can differentiate fact from feeling, it puts distance between you and the event. It lets you take yourself and your feelings out of the picture. It gives you a chance to take "time out" and to see what is happening.

> *God, grant me the Serenity to accept*
> *the things I cannot change . . .*
> *Courage to change the things I can . . .*
> *and Wisdom to know the difference . . .*
> —Reinhold Niebuhr

5. *Handle Anger and Guilt*

What do you do when the responsibilities of caregiving become such an emotional burden that you resent the time you spend with the person with dementia? How do you handle your anger with others at home or at work, who you believe don't understand? Feelings of anger and then guilt that enter into your thoughts again and again diminish your spirit. Instead of depleting your strength, try to turn your anger and guilt into something positive for yourself.

- Tell your family and colleagues that you are going through a very difficult period right now. You only have so much energy and much of it is being given to the person affected with Alzheimer's disease or related dementia.
- Don't go it alone. Tell your family and colleagues that you are having difficulty adjusting your priorities and that you need help in sorting them out. Others will have some good ideas because they have gone through this before, or are going through it right now. Create a support group for yourself or attend a support group already in progress through the Alzheimer's Association.
- Admit you cannot be at the "top of your game" all the time.
- Try not to expect too much of yourself. Be gentle with yourself.
- Find someone with whom you can "blow off steam" and laugh. Tell your best friend what you are feeling and laugh at yourself for taking yourself too seriously.
- Try some physical exercise. Walk each day for 20 to 30 minutes. Help your body release some of the pent up emotions.
- Forgive yourself. Try to be understanding of other people's needs and your own needs. Say your favorite prayer of forgiveness. "I confess to your blessings upon me, and I confess to you my sins, so forgive me." (Muslim) "Forgive us our trespasses as we forgive those who trespass against us . . ." (Christian)

Anyone can become angry. That is easy. But to be angry
with the right person, to the right degree, at the right time,
for the right reason and in the right way—that is not easy.
— Aristotle

6. *Find Ways to Relax . . . And Discipline Yourself to Do Them*

- Work in the yard or your garden;
- Take a walk or run to renew your body;
- Get ready for bed in a leisurely way;

- Place a rocking chair in a special place and surround it with only good books and magazines—or things that please you;
- Take up a sport with friends: golf, bowling, racquetball, etc.;
- Walk your neighbor's dog or yours and enjoy the scenery;
- Enjoy cooking a meal for friends;
- Draw or paint for half an hour a day;
- Make music or listen to music on the way home from work, rather than the news;
- Ride your motorcycle into the hills alone or with friends;
- Get a massage.

Try this:
- Take "minute vacations" by picturing yourself in your favorite place (actual or not).
- Hang pictures on your walls at home and at the office to remind yourself of your special place or special people in your life.
- At the beginning of the day, think about what is ahead for you, your family, your work, your caregiving. Block out 15 to 30 minutes just for you. Keep a date with yourself and spend those minutes freely as you wish.
- If you keep a "To Do" list, make sure that you and your needs are on the top of the list. Discipline yourself to do something to relax each day.

You will be an emotionally stronger spouse, parent, friend, and caregiver if you systematically take care of your physical, emotional, intellectual, and spiritual self.

> *Too much of a good thing can be wonderful.*
> —Mae West

7. Keep Friends Close; They Will Give You Energy to Keep Going

As you come to be more involved in caregiving, the tendency is to let go of your friends when work and family responsibilities become too burdensome. It is common for the caregiver to put himself or herself last. Typically she or he performs the duties of a parent, a spouse, a worker outside the home, a son or daughter, and a caregiver. The caregiver's inner self becomes neglected. Current literature tells us that caregivers need friends to help nurture the person inside.

"A landmark UCLA study suggests friendships between women are special. They shape who we are and who we are yet to be. They soothe our tumultuous inner world, fill the emotional gaps in our marriage, and help us remember who we really are. By the way, they may do even more. Scientists now suspect that hanging out with our friends can actually counteract the kind of stomach quivering stress most of us experience on a daily basis . . ." From UCLA Study on Friendship Among Women by Gale Berkowitz.

☙ Share humor with friends. Example: "Hi, Marie, how was your dad today?" "Pretty good," Marie answers, "but I spent most of my time looking for dad's bottom teeth. I looked everywhere: under the bed, in the closet, the kitchen, etc. I think he wore them once and then threw them out. Just one of those normal days . . ."
☙ Share sorrow with friends. Example: Here is a note written by a person who just lost her good friend. Notice how she asks for what she needs from her friends.

"It is with a heavy heart that I tell you that Ellen died at noon, Thursday, of a massive heart attack. I can't even begin to express my grief at her passing. The void she will leave will be huge and right now I'm not doing very well with her death. I am asking all of you to come to my aid and make sure I get a good belly laugh in her honor. (Wait at least one week, please.)"

You may forget with whom you laughed,
but you will never forget with whom you wept.
—Arab Proverb

8. Be Responsible vs. Responsive

The stages of Alzheimer's disease will determine when it is time to be sympathetic and receptive to the requests of the person and when it is time to be accountable for his or her actions.

For example: When Joe, a person in the early stages of Alzheimer's disease, still wants to drive the car and does so safely, you can easily go for a ride with him and even let him go for a drive alone. When Joe says, "Let's go to the store," you can willingly ride along.

However, when Joe gets lost while driving, parks the car, and then cannot find it, his dementia is progressing. He should not continue to drive because he could do harm to others and himself.

When the person continually asks to have the car keys—and even gets very angry with you—as a caregiver you need to be "responsible" and find ways to keep the person from driving.

Here is an example of how this situation was solved by one family:

Joe insists repeatedly that he can drive the car. This nagging overwhelms the family members and they have no choice but to pretend that the car has been stolen. At the same time they have friends who are sympathetic to their needs. The family reports the car stolen. One of the friends comes to the home and tells Joe that the car has been stolen and that it cannot be found.

Joe knows the family friend and accepts the news. He stops asking for the keys because a family member told him another car cannot be purchased. Joe is satisfied.

Peace returned to Joe and his family.

> *Have patience with all things,*
> *but first of all with yourself.*
> —St. Francis de Sales

9. Accept Life's Frailties

- It is very hard for the healthy and young to accept illness. Sometimes it is a burden on the whole family to visit the sick. When the family is centered solely on the needs of the one who is frail, there can be problems. When Sunday becomes *the* day to visit, it can become a day that is resented by everyone in the family. So what do you do?
- Let go of the idea that everyone needs to be a caregiver. As the disease progresses, not everyone can handle the discomfort and stress of seeing a loved one's health diminish. The caregiver should be perceptive and not make everyone in the family participate all the time.
- The caregiver should be sensitive to individuals with Alzheimer's disease who can no longer tolerate a large number of visitors. As the disease progresses, it is difficult for the loved one to handle a lot of stimulation—more than one or two people visiting, the TV turned on, pets running around—all at the same time. Visits don't need to be long. Not more than one or two people should be taking the attention of the person at any one time. Look for the quality of time in your interactions, not the quantity of time or number of people involved.
- Make special time for everyone in the family—the healthy and the sick. Celebrate the lives of all family members; don't let the person who is ill dominate your thoughts and actions.
- Get help from the Alzheimer's Association with their support groups, respite care opportunities, and other programs.

*Illness is the night-side of life, a more onerous
citizenship. Everyone who is born holds dual
citizenship, in the kingdom of the well and in the
kingdom of the sick. Although we all prefer to
use only the good passport, sooner or later each
of us is obligated, at least for a spell, to identify
ourselves as citizens of that other place.*

—Susan Sontag

10. Reflect on a "Patient's Bill of Rights"

Reflect on how you—as a caregiver—are helping your loved one live the most productive life possible. Give yourself credit for all the things you are doing for your loved one.

Patient's Bill of Rights

Every person diagnosed with Alzheimer's disease or a related disorder deserves:

- To be informed of one's diagnosis
- To have appropriate, ongoing medical care
- To be productive in work and play as long as possible
- To be treated like an adult, not like a child
- To have expressed feelings taken seriously
- To be free from psychotropic medication if at all possible
- To live in a safe, structured and predictable environment
- To enjoy meaningful activities to fill each day
- To be out-of-doors on a regular basis
- To have physical contact including hugging, caressing, and hand-holding
- To be with persons who know one's life story, including cultural and religious traditions
- To be cared for by individuals well-trained in dementia care

(Developed by: Virginia March Bell, MSW, Alzheimer's Association, Lexington/Bluegrass Chapter Kentucky; David Troxel, MPH, Alzheimer's Association, Santa Barbara Chapter, California)

*Life is what we make it, always has been,
always will be.*

—Grandma Moses

11. *Create Your Personal "Advisory Board"*

When tough decisions need to be made, read some information available on the topic, and talk with as many people as you can who have been in similar situations. But go a step farther—create your own personal "Advisory Board" composed of people from the present and the past. Choose five or six people for specific qualities you admire to sit at your imaginary table. People whose methods or styles of communicating are different from your own make excellent board members.

In your mind, picture a round table. You are sitting with people like:

- Your great aunt who has a lot of wisdom;
- Your eighth grade teacher who had common sense about important issues;
- Your pastor, priest, rabbi, minister, or spiritual leader who influenced you the most;
- Your closest friend who understands you and the many dimensions of your current situation;
- A person who always challenges you to think "out of the box;"
- A doctor who knows about Alzheimer's disease and related dementia.

Place before your imaginary Advisory Board the simple and more complex daily decisions you need to make on behalf of the person with dementia. You may find your situations are much like those found in the stories in Part III.

Your imaginary Advisory Board will always suggest three ways of responding in each situation. As you make decisions, you will notice patterns emerging. As the disease progresses, you will see how your style will change to meet the needs of the person who has Alzheimer's disease or related dementia.

You will become more comfortable in your role as caregiver. You will have prayed for guidance, sought information from professionals, consulted with other family members, and reflected on what your Advisory Board might advise. You can move forward, confident that you have done all you can and make the decisions that seem appropriate.

> *No one gets up in the morning and says, 'Today I am going to make the worst decision I can.' Decisions are made with the best of intentions. Some turn out to be great; others turn out to be faulty. We do the best we can.*
> —Bill Flynn, Spouse of a Caregiver

12. *Nurture What Remains*

Over the years of being a caregiver, the tip to "nurture what remains," has been the most helpful for me. Take time to think about this "tip" and you will be greatly rewarded. Families who have had someone diagnosed with Alzheimer's disease carry with them the burden of knowing there is no cure at this time.

Some researchers are challenging many assumptions that have been held about the disease.

Some studies are challenging old theories about the sense of personhood among those diagnosed with dementia. "Giving Voice to Persons Living with Dementia: The Researcher's Opportunities and Challenges" by Jane Hollet and Theresa Moore, and the study "Self-Consciousness and Alzheimer's Disease" by Roger Gil, et al. give new insights into the capabilities for introspection remaining in persons with Alzheimer's disease as well as other significant findings.

As research continues on the study of the inner world and consciousness of persons with dementia, caregivers, family members, and friends will have more opportunities to explore new ways to live and work with those affected with the disease.

In Part V of this handbook Roger A. Brumback talks about both the *medical* treatment of Alzheimer's disease and the *supportive* treatment of Alzheimer's disease. This *supportive* treatment involves "the education of the affected individual, caregivers, family, and friends regarding both the lost and the preserved brain functions. . . . Instead of focusing on deficits, the focus should be on the preserved abilities and the development of compensatory strategies," according to Roger A. Brumback.

Caregivers generally need time to process new knowledge about the disease. In the process of thinking about and discussing the new knowledge, understanding can result. When caregivers understand what is happening to the person who has the disease, they can become more compassionate and are able to find new ways to provide the best care possible. Many caregivers will be able to relate to Part II of this handbook.

The chart at the end of this section, "A Caregiver's Perspective: Preserved Skills That Can Be Nourished During Disease Progression," is based on the experiences of one of the authors (Pat Callone) of being a caregiver to three family members who have or have had Alzheimer's disease. The chart highlights what can be experienced at different stages of the disease. The search for preserved abilities is very rewarding and can lead both the caregiver and the person being cared for to new dimensions of understanding each other.

Based on your own experiences—as a caregiver, family member, or friend of a person with Alzheimer's disease or related dementia—you can develop your own chart about what is happening with your loved one during the progression of the disease. Through discussion and reflection on what is happening, you will be rewarded with a certain joy in knowing you are doing what is life-giving to your loved one. The unique personhood of those with the disease remains and can be stimulated and nourished throughout all the stages of the disease.

Part V of this handbook describes the progression of Alzheimer's disease and related dementia. Understanding the physical course of the disease can help in understanding family members diagnosed with the disease and what is happening in their brains as the disease progresses. Expectations became more realistic and less demanding.

When reviewed in light of the Caregiver's Perspective chart on page 25, these facts may be helpful to you as caregiver, family member, or friend of persons with Alzheimer's disease or related dementia. The caregiving experience—although rigorous—has its own unique rewards.

About Dementia

- Dementia is not really a disease, but is a symptom of something going wrong in the brain. In other words, dementia is what you witness in the patient's behavior, but what is happening in the brain is the disease causing the dementia.
- Sometimes the disease causing dementia is actually a treatable condition. On the other hand, some causes of dementia are irreversible and ultimately fatal because the nerve cells in the brain die.
- The brain is different from other organs of the body in that every nerve cell in the brain does something unique which only that nerve cell can do and no other nerve cell can do.
- In the brain, every part has a specific function, and all the parts must work together for the brain to work correctly. Loss of any part of the brain results in loss of that function, because no other part of the brain can take over or perform that function.
- Alzheimer's disease causes the progressive death of nerve cells.

During the early-to-mild stage of Alzheimer's disease (generally a 3- to 5-year period), the following changes occur:

- The memory area of the brain is the first area in which nerve cells die as a result of Alzheimer's disease.
- Because judgment, reasoning, and social skills are still functioning normally, the person can develop compensatory coping strategies to deal with the memory problems.
- Thus, in the beginning stage of the disease process, no one will be aware of the problem because of these compensations, and the person will often appear normal and never consult a physician.

As the disease progresses toward the moderate stage of Alzheimer's (generally a 3- to-5 year period), more changes occur:

- The wave of destruction spreads. At this stage, the individual has

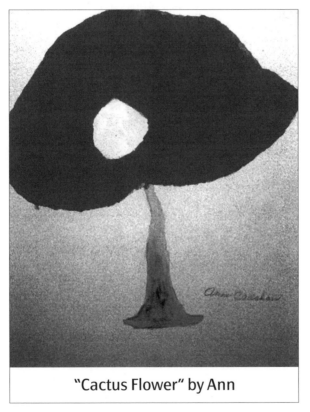

"Cactus Flower" by Ann

Ann was born in the Midwest. Her painting depicts the simplicity of nature. In the Memories in the Making art program, every picture has value. The ensuing sense of accomplishment brings renewed joy and self-respect to the person with the disease.

trouble dressing, gets lost or disoriented, and cannot figure out how to use objects.

✦ This is also the stage of the disease process during which driving becomes problematic because the individual cannot integrate all the visual and audible information of the environment with the proper body sensations of the steering wheel and floor pedals.

✦ During this time patients generally consult physicians for evaluation. Family members and acquaintances become aware that a problem requiring medical evaluation exists.

As the disease progresses into the severe stage of Alzheimer's disease, the following changes occur:

✦ The person loses the ability to interact properly. At this stage, many patients can no longer be managed at home by caregivers. The person loses judgment, reasoning, and social skills.

✦ Because the median survival (the time by which half of Alzheimer's patients die) is 7 years after diagnosis, many individuals will die before they reach the severe stage of the disease.

✦ Survival during the severe stage depends a lot on the quality of nursing care because patients lose many of the self-care functions that prevent other illnesses. Alzheimer's disease is the underlying cause of death; that is, it weakens the brain's control of body systems and allows other illnesses to end the patient's life.

A CAREGIVER'S PERSPECTIVE

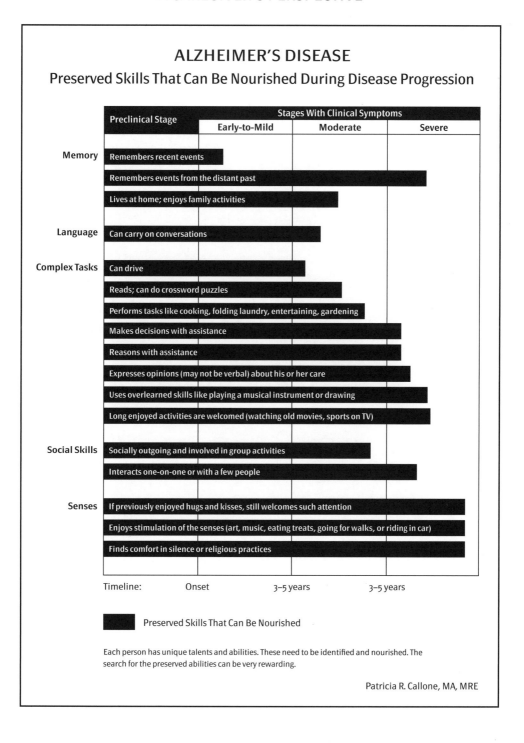

ALZHEIMER'S DISEASE
Preserved Skills That Can Be Nourished During Disease Progression

	Preclinical Stage	Stages With Clinical Symptoms		
		Early-to-Mild	Moderate	Severe
Memory	Remembers recent events			
	Remembers events from the distant past			
	Lives at home; enjoys family activities			
Language	Can carry on conversations			
Complex Tasks	Can drive			
	Reads; can do crossword puzzles			
	Performs tasks like cooking, folding laundry, entertaining, gardening			
	Makes decisions with assistance			
	Reasons with assistance			
	Expresses opinions (may not be verbal) about his or her care			
	Uses overlearned skills like playing a musical instrument or drawing			
	Long enjoyed activities are welcomed (watching old movies, sports on TV)			
Social Skills	Socially outgoing and involved in group activities			
	Interacts one-on-one or with a few people			
Senses	If previously enjoyed hugs and kisses, still welcomes such attention			
	Enjoys stimulation of the senses (art, music, eating treats, going for walks, or riding in car)			
	Finds comfort in silence or religious practices			

Timeline: Onset   3–5 years   3–5 years

■ Preserved Skills That Can Be Nourished

Each person has unique talents and abilities. These need to be identified and nourished. The search for the preserved abilities can be very rewarding.

Patricia R. Callone, MA, MRE

The Reluctant Caregiver: A Husband And Wife's Personal Story

Meet Carl J. Pfeifer, D Min and Janaan Manternach, D Min

anaan and I met at The Catholic University of America. Both of us were students in the Religious Education Department. She was also working on a religion curriculum at what was then known as the Confraternity of Christian Doctrine Office. I became interested in what she was doing, because I was experiencing little success teaching religion to 4th graders at St. Anthony's Parish in Northeast Washington. She gave me some rules and teaching suggestions that I followed, and they worked. She, in turn, asked me to read lesson plans that she was writing and, eventually, I was asked to join the staff to work with her and do other writing at the Confraternity of Christian Doctrine office.

It had never been my intention to write curriculum for children. My goal was to return to St. Louis and teach at the University. However, I discovered in myself a gift for writing curriculum and for creating supportive materials for catechists and religion teachers. I found also that my theological and biblical training was a perfect match with Janaan's practical, poetic, and creative teaching skills. Besides that, both of us wrote easily and enjoyed doing it.

I was always interested in photography and was responsible for introducing photos into our religion textbooks.

Because of our work at the Confraternity and the creation of textbooks, we had many opportunities to lecture, teach, and conduct workshops. I enjoyed addressing groups and, although shy, perhaps because I prepared carefully, I could do it with ease.

One of the greatest blessings in Janaan's and my life are our godchildren, Angela and Miguel Barbieri. They have taught us what it means to love unconditionally. They have filled our home with laughter and have shown us, experientially, what it is like to be a child, a teen, and now young adults. Best of all, they care not a wit that I have Alzheimer's. They love me now, as they always have—just as I am.

(*Statement directed by Carl.*)

Meet Janaan Manternach, D Min

I was never interested in Alzheimer's disease. I knew it was out there messing up people's lives, but no one I knew had been diagnosed with it. It's true that Carl's Mom suffered from what her physician diagnosed as a deterioration of the cells at the base of her brain, but he insisted it was not Alzheimer's disease. Now, Carl and I are not sure!

We now wonder if there is a genetic link, but since we don't have children of our own, that question, for us, is mostly moot. What isn't moot is that Carl has the disease, and it is forcing both of us, especially me, to do what we can to make a difference in what happens about the disease in the future. As changes occur in Carl, I find myself asking questions: "How can I fine tune my responses so that his new needs are met and his spirit is enhanced? Will what I'm doing work?"

During our active professional lives, we wrote articles, columns, and books—mostly for catechists and religion teachers. We lectured extensively throughout the United States and Europe. It seems a bit ironic to us now that a key ingredient in all our writings was life experience. Through this prism, we tried to help the learner discern truth and wisdom and insight to be more than they were at the moment. Carl and I find ourselves doing something of the same on a daily basis as we cope with Alzheimer's disease. This is why our first attempt at making a difference is through writing a chapter for this book. We have this opportunity because Barbara Vasiloff, one of the other authors, invited us to do it. She was an able assistant to us in Washington, D.C. We have remained close friends and are profoundly inspired by her work, Discipline with Purpose.

She was one of the first persons that we told that Carl suffers from the disease and, with her support during the last three years, I've come to the realization that I have moved from a temporary caregiver to a permanent one. During that time, Carl and I have asked ourselves many questions, both silently and aloud. As we grappled with our changing relationship and sought ways to keep dignity and purpose in our lives, some answers were found. Our questions continue to evolve, as do our answers. These twelve questions and the answers we are living with are offered to you, the reader, to help you in your journey.

You will recognize the characteristics of the early-to-mild stage of Alzheimer's disease as we sought to understand what was happening to Carl. Many of the dozen tips for caregivers that are listed in Part I of this book are helpful things I have done to keep my own spirit alive. I am beginning to recognize when I must change from my preferred way of interacting with Carl to a caregiving style that better meets his needs. I often review Dr. Brumback's information about what the disease is doing to Carl's brain, and it helps to remind me that in spite of the functions being lost, much will remain even into the severe stage of the disease. I also keep returning to Pat Callone's chart, "Preserved Skills That Can Be Nourished during Disease Progression" and to Dr. Brumback's "Timeline of Preserved Skills in Stages of Disease Progression." Both of them not only specifically identify what functions are affected by the disease, but also indicate how long the person with dementia may be able to reasonably function in the use of each one.

As a writer, I have a passion to use the written and spoken word to reveal hidden facets of reality. I am beginning to believe that what is happening to Carl and me is not an accident. Carl is co-author of this material with me. We have discussed all twelve of the questions I have as a caregiver. Together, we share this special journey of our life together in our mid-seventies.

It is a challenge to continue using our gifts in honest and inspiring ways so that others—on the same journey—can find their way happily and peacefully to not only survive, but also to grow wiser because of it.

TWELVE QUESTIONS AND ANSWERS

Q: How do I balance my identity as wife and caregiver?

A: This is tricky. Identifying oneself as a "caregiver" can be a monumental challenge. Admittedly, I resisted the whole idea as long as I could, because the role does not come naturally to me.

In the past when Carl had surgery or was temporarily sick—with the flu or an asthma attack—I would tell him, partly in jest but mostly meaning it, that I would only give him one or two days of tender loving care. After that he was on his own. Yet, "caregiving" has always been a part of the loving relationship between us. We have both done it for each other; however, Carl has always been much better at it than I. His concern, when I was ill or recovering from surgery, was to help me get better no matter how long it took or what it did to his schedule.

I'm aware now that I have gradually gone from hoping that my caregiving role would be temporary to knowing it is one of a permanent caregiver. As the change to permanent caregiver took place in me, I took out on Carl the anger I was feeling over the loss of my independence and the limitations we were experiencing. Because of that, I've come up with some "perhapses."

- ❧ Perhaps it is best to wear the "caregiver" identity lightly until, in the day-to-day living with the person with dementia, you grow into a realization of what it means. There will be small and bigger signs, like needing to help tie shoelaces, button the cuffs of a shirt, take care of medication, and do most of the driving. As each of these things occur, the identity of "caregiver" becomes more real.
- ❧ Perhaps you should carefully hold on to your identity as husband, wife, son, or daughter by not allowing the demands of caregiver to diminish your desire to socialize with friends, continue to read, write, hold down a job, take care of a family, whatever. . . . Interestingly, I've found that the more I continue to do what I can do apart from caregiving, the less my husband's diminishments erode my spirit and time. However, I'm realistic enough to accept the truth that the demands will increase and that adjustments will have to be made.

I believe that protecting our identity apart from that of "caregiver" can also protect the dignity and essence of the person with Alzheimer's disease. To care too much too early could hasten losses. I refuse to do what I hope Carl can do, and I allow him to struggle more than he might. In doing this, I've found that he wants to continue being involved in all aspects of life.

Part of the struggle is being willing to accept the losses in the person with dementia and respond with care and kindness. I don't want Carl to be less than he has been because it dramatically affects who we are as a couple, as friends and lovers. I hate it with my whole being. In spite of that, I'm gradually beginning to accept what he can't change and am learning to appreciate the less in him than the more I long for.

Q: How do I handle being constantly interrupted?

A: Initially, and for a fairly long period of time, I became angry when Carl came into my office with a question or for help in finding something. Sometimes he would just come into my space and stand there. The latter was particularly annoying.

My anger was expressed in unkind words like, "You don't have anything you have to do so please let me get something done." Or, "Don't stand over me like that." I really wanted him and his disease out of my sight. I was totally unwilling to stop what I was doing to deal with what I considered "inconsequential needs." I felt that the least he could do was to give me space to accomplish something.

I'm a bit ashamed of my behavior, but now when I'm working at my computer, he rarely disturbs me. So perhaps, for now, the dynamic was not all bad.

Caregiving does not, I believe, necessarily mean that you are at the person with Alzheimer's disease constant beck and call. In the later stages of the disease, that may be necessary, but in the early and moderate stages, I believe that it is wise to call upon him or her to function as fully as possible. That being said, I'm becoming less selfish and more adaptable, which seems to give my husband the security and protection he needs to allow me to work for good lengths of time without interruption.

Q: How can I strengthen my resolve to take the time to listen when my husband is trying to communicate, in order to give him the dignity he deserves?

A: Since I am internally programmed to "hurry," this is something that is unusually hard for me. Whenever Carl is in my presence, it is normal for him to want to say something. He knows what he wants to say, begins to speak, but is often only able to utter one word. Baffled and frustrated, he struggles to communicate. I ask questions or make suggestions, hoping to help him bring order to the incoherence he's experiencing, but all too quickly I tell him. "It's okay, not to worry."

Actually, I don't want to take the time to help him find a way to communicate what he needs to tell or wants to say. I've kind of gotten into a pattern of dismissing his attempts, and he has gotten into a pattern of giving up. It's only very recently that I'm becoming aware of this as wrong-headed, selfish, uncaring, and perhaps even hastening the loss of his ability to share what is going on and to keep alive his verbal skills.

One of the steps we now take to free him to communicate is to go to lunch together, and in that setting, spontaneously talk. I ask questions. He answers as fully as he can. He makes observations. We comment on the food, and he always wants to know where we're going next. Never does he have difficulty phrasing that last question.

Another thing that I do is talk to myself about slowing down enough to willingly listen when he has the urge to communicate. Deep down, I know that I don't want to lose any of what he still has to say, nor do I want him to stop exercising his mind with words and sentences. I'm also keenly aware that good listening means we stop what we're doing, clear our mental and physical distractions, and focus on the person. We listen to their words and to the underlying message that only our hearts can hear. I believe, too, that this might be the most sacred moment Carl and I will have in our day and that this positive act of listening is a gift we give to each other.

Still another way that we've found that frees up his flow of language is to share impressions about a show or newscast that we're watching on television. I also read aloud to him and invite him to react.

Finally, one of the best ways, so far, is to get together, at least once weekly, with friends who talk directly to him; not just to me, and who help him to be an equal participant in our conversations.

I think, as caregivers, we can unwittingly hasten losses, and I believe that if we hasten the loss of speech, we not only risk isolating the person with dementia from himself but also from ourselves and others.

All too soon, the disease will rob the person of normal ways of communicating, but until that time, we need to keep strengthening our resolve to help him or her bring order out of words in chaos and to hold on to thoughts that, with a vengeance, try to slip away.

Q: What strategies can I use to enable my husband to be ready to go somewhere within a certain time frame?

A: My initial strategy was screaming at Carl when he wasn't ready to leave after I had forewarned him about the time we needed to go. I still get impatient when he has had several reminders and is still not ready to leave when it's time.

I find that I constantly have to work on strategies because reminders don't seem to work. Some that I'm working on are:

- Show him the appointment on our calendar and indicate the time we need to leave. This may have to be done several times prior to leaving.

- A half hour before it's time to leave, I remind him that he has to change clothes or do whatever he needs to do to be ready. If it's a matter of changing clothes, he may need more time.
- Fifteen, ten, and five minutes before it's time to leave, I ask him if he's ready and/or if he needs help to get ready.
- My most successful strategy is to leave the house with plenty of time to get where we need to go, even if we anticipate an appointment by 20 to 30 minutes.

This may not be a challenge for all caregivers. I think it depends on a readiness style prior to the disease. Carl, for as long as I have known him, was never in a hurry to go any place, and I have exercised a constant impatience with his unreadiness. The disease has simply exaggerated this pattern.

As with the other challenges aforementioned, I find that, as a caregiver, I need to be supportive of him, no matter what!

Q: How can we become comfortable telling others openly and freely that my loved one has Alzheimer's disease?

A: Initially, we weren't comfortable at all. We were in deep denial and didn't mention it. Others were aware that something was going on, however, but they didn't mention it either. Our first step to acceptance and acknowledgment started with an appointment with a neurologist. He, on the other hand, was sure that Carl's history of depression was the cause of his memory lapses. At that time, Carl's speech wasn't affected, and he continued to work. He scored high on tests he was given to evaluate his mental acumen, and an MRI indicated that his brain appeared normal. Yet, his ability to lecture was falling apart, and his memory was beginning to betray him more and more.

We then began to see psychiatrists who were recommended to us, and after time with four of them, we were still without a diagnosis. We had come to our own conclusion that something was truly going awry in his brain, however, and we began telling our family, friends, and others, when the need arose, that Carl was experiencing "severe memory loss."

When he began having difficulty conversing, unable to find the words he needed to express his thoughts, we began to own up to the possibility that he had Alzheimer's disease. Since then, we are both open and comfortable with naming the disease. However, I couldn't stop there.

One thing that I began to do assiduously, after reading the introduction to Pat Callone's chapter, was to read everything that I could about the disease. For example:

- *Losing My Mind: An Intimate Look at Life with Alzheimer's* (2002) and *When It Gets Dark: An Enlightened Reflection on Life with Alzheimer's* (2003), both by Thomas De Baggio. Free Press, A Division of Simon & Schuster
- *Through the Wilderness of Alzheimer's, A Guide in Two Voices* by Robert and Anne Simpson. Augsburg Fortress, 1999
- *The Memory Bible* by Gary Small, M.D. Hyperion Books, 2002
- *Aging with Grace* by David Snowdon, Ph.D. Bantam Books, 2001
- *The Forgetting: Alzheimer's Portrait of an Epidemic* by David Shenk. Anchor Books, 2002
- *Alzheimer's: The Complete Guide to Proofing Your Home* by Mark L. Warner. Purdue University Press, 2000

These and other books have been recommended to us, and I plan to read them too. And, although expensive ($195 for one year), we have subscribed to the John Hopkins Memory Bulletin (P. O. Box 420880, Palm Coast, FL 32142-9616).

I've also been toying with setting aside fifteen minutes a day to pray, to calm and ready myself for what each new day might bring. My husband regularly gives hints of losses as he experiences them; however, he really doesn't know what's going on. Often when I ask him how he's doing he says, "I really don't know."

Continuing to participate in social situations, keeping in close touch with friends and family, and repeatedly telling him that I love him, to which he responds in kind, help to enhance and protect his dignity. One thing that is becoming clear is that we can't do this alone. The more we develop an acceptance of the disease, the less shame we experience, and the more we share, the more support we receive.

Q: How can I mature into a willingness to do what needs to be done to protect and enhance my loved one's dignity?

A: This is an ongoing process. Anger continues to have a hold on me because I repeatedly find myself unwilling to reckon with the things Carl forgets—like putting things away, taking his medicine when I put it out, and other routine, seemingly mindless actions.

I keep telling myself after these situations repeatedly occur that he simply doesn't remember; however, it is also after I've yelled at him or expressed unhappiness at his behavior. He seems to realize that I'm merely acting out of frustration, yet I know that it has to add to the misery he is going through as he keeps losing more and more of himself.

As I've wondered and commiserated about my anger at the disease, I'm beginning to realize that over the years of marriage (27 for us) a oneness occurs and that I'm not only losing the vibrant, brilliant, loving, and caring person that I married, I'm also losing part of myself. In the wake of that, loneliness and helplessness wash over me and depression dances at the edges of my consciousness.

In spite of the anger, frustration, and occasional loneliness, I know deep down—and I hang on to the belief—that he will be able to depend on my love for him and that I will be the support that he needs.

I read with interest Barb Vasiloff's three caregiving styles outlined in this book. I've never had trouble knowing myself nor the way I prefer to respond and interact with others. In many situations, however, my preferred style no longer works for me or for my husband. When I deliberately select another style of communicating and change my perspective to meet his ever changing needs, things seem to click. I know now I am the one who must do the changing.

Q: How do I reckon with the fact that my constant concern and preoccupation with the vagaries of the disease keep me in a constant need of more rest?

A: I reckon with it by owning up to the fact that I'm caught in a situation that isn't going to get better and will gradually worsen. I'm keenly aware that the weariness I feel is mostly caused by the heaviness of the burden that Alzheimer's disease places on both Carl and me, even when there are times during each day when its demands aren't operative.

I also have a growing awareness that the disease—because it is irreversible and progressive— is like a battering ram against hope. This, at times, really saps my energy. I have learned to take restorative measures, like going for a walk together, preparing a special meal, playing solitaire while he sits nearby watching television, or I read a book or listen to music while he sits in a chair and sleeps.

I have not yet found a way to deal with the restlessness I regularly experience at night when I'm trying to sleep. Sometimes, before I go to sleep, an emptiness engulfs me, and I find myself crying. Sleep seemingly is easier for me in the morning, so I sleep longer then. And, when I do get up I'm refreshed enough to feel happy about the new day and its possibilities and challenges. It's at that time, too, that I remember anew what I deeply believe: "That God is with and for us all the time. We are not alone."

Ritual is another thing that helps my husband and me cope. We eat breakfast every day, pretty much at the same time, except on Sundays when we go to church and eat breakfast afterwards. He sets the table for dinner in the evening, does the dishes afterwards, and takes out the garbage. He not only does these things effortlessly, he wants to do them. That eases my resentment about a lot of the things that he can no longer do and gives me some peace.

We purposely get out of the house every day for a change of scenery. We go to lunch, or to a grocery store or the cleaners, or to a book or video store. Doctor appointments also take us out fairly regularly. And, we now attend, more frequently, evening and afternoon events at our Church, which are noted in the Sunday Bulletin. These, though very ordinary activities, are usually restful, even fun. We are usually conversing during these forays and sometimes something happens that makes it all worthwhile. I asked him one day while we were eating lunch, "What makes you happy?" Without hesitating a moment he answered, "YOU".

Restlessness is essentially a product of worry, and I haven't yet found ways to escape the pain that I feel at the loss of sparkle in his eyes and the worry that overtakes me at other losses in him that become regularly apparent. So far, I reckon with what is, and most of the time I'm tired.

Q: What do I do with the guilt I feel when my responses are genuinely non-caring or reveal a denial of what is happening in the person I'm caring for?

A: I keep forgiving myself and him. I sometimes tell Carl, "I'm sorry!" but I don't do that very often, perhaps not often enough. He frequently shows me, in his own way, that he regrets what's happening.

There's a mystery in the progression of the disease that keeps both of us a bit off balance. The limitations that are part of this progression, in him, show up in the most ordinary circumstances. For example:

- He's often unable to find the *TV Guide* or the remote control, although they have, for years, been in the same place.
- Or, many times he can't put the pages of a newspaper back together after reading it.
- Or, he doesn't remember the simplest sequence of events and needs to be reminded over and over.

➤ And, although we watch the same newscasts in the evening, he consistently worries that I won't turn to the right channel.

These are just a few of the losses that occur daily, and they could seem petty and inconsequential, yet they aren't. New ones occur with regularity, and they add up to a lot of pain. It's at these times when I realize how much I hate what's happening and, admittedly, I express my distress in outrage, mostly low-level, but outrage, nonetheless. This, I believe, is not only forgivable, but normal.

I've found, also, that expressing frustration doesn't necessarily hurt but can be helpful to the person with Alzheimer's disease. For example, I was genuinely distressed when Carl, in urinating, splashed urine on the floor around the stool. With anger, I insisted that he clean it up and told him exactly what do to. He followed my directions and has taken care of the problem ever since.

Many caregivers, in situations like mine, handle the everyday challenges with much more patience and nobility than I. I'm filled with admiration for them. What's happening between us seems to be working, however, and I'm keenly aware that I won't give up on either myself or Carl. Right now, we have no other choice but to keep muddling through, loving each other, and forgiving each other as best we can.

Q: How do I keep loving the person who is, in many ways, no longer the spouse I fell in love with?

A: This, to some extent, takes an act of will. Since "for better or worse" was not a part of our marriage vows, I don't consider that as something that is binding me now. When I married my husband, however, I knew in my whole being that it was forever. And, that is binding!

As with so much that is part of the disease of Alzheimer's, there is mystery to the loving that continues between a couple when one of them, in many ways, is slowly becoming a different partner.

When I look into my husband's eyes and see a dullness, a lack of sparkle, it's like a blow to my spirit. Since our conversations are now pretty much limited to — "How are you doing?", "What are you thinking now?", "How are you feeling?", "What makes you happy?", "Where are we going next?", or "What are we doing tomorrow?"—I experience a loneliness and hunger for the spirited conversations, arguments, and lengthy discussions we used to have. Yet, those losses don't seem to disturb my love for him at all.

Throughout our marriage, we said to each other daily, "I love you!" These were never empty words, even when we were angry with one another. We continue to do that today, except we seem to do it more often. Most of the time, in the past, I was the initiator in these daily affirmations of affection. Today, he initiates them more, and I find healing in the truth that he continues to consciously and actively love me.

I'm learning that part of what it means to go on this journey with Carl is to never give up on him or myself. I often feel sorrow, I often wonder "Why?", I often get scared of what lies ahead, and I often plead with God, Mary, and the Saints to heal him. To admit to praying like that embarrasses me a bit, yet I can't stop doing it.

An important reality in the art of continuing to love Carl is the knowledge that he profoundly needs me, too. And, in many ways, I also need him to continue loving me.

Finally, I could never have imagined what it would be like to have this disease in our marriage, and it is continually forcing me to be creative in its management. Likewise, I cannot imagine ever not loving Carl so that is, I believe, another invitation to greater creativity.

Q: How do we deal with social situations in which the person with Alzheimer's disease can't participate?

A: I find this so painful that I have sometimes wondered about curtailing our social life. To begin with, Carl has always been shy and has never been overly talkative in social situations. He was keenly alert to conversations and to what was going on, however, and he actively participated when he was invited to or felt a need to agree, disagree, or add his own insights.

That ability is pretty much gone now. He often sits within a group and says nothing. And sometimes, he simply falls asleep. The latter, I believe, is one way of surviving amidst a group that is supposedly functioning normally.

I have tried, at times, to clue him in to what is being said, but this makes him uncomfortable when he doesn't readily understand, and attention is drawn to him. Often, I simply reach for his hand and hold it for a while. He responds to this, and it seems to make us both feel better.

Even though I tell him several times before we go to a party, a dinner, or other gathering, he often doesn't remember until it's time to get ready and to leave. If we're going to a close friend's home, he's happy to go, but if it's a larger gathering, I notice a hesitancy and a bit of fear when he finds out where we're going. On the other hand, if it's a reception or party for one of his colleagues or friends, he enjoys being a part of it and remarks about how good it was when we get home. I have learned that it's important to never leave him by himself in social settings. If I need to leave him briefly, I tell him where to wait for me and that, so far, works out well.

We have to send regrets, at times, and every time we do, I experience a new kind of loneliness. We've also curtailed the work conventions we used to attend. This has been especially hard, because they've always been energizing and learning events for me. This has taken us "out of the loop" so to speak.

The most I can say at this point in our dealing with the disease is that we need to be with others. Social situations greatly ease the burden.

Q: What do I do with the resentment I feel about having to take over all the tasks and jobs that used to be my loved one's responsibilities?

A: I used to grumble about it and frequently vented my resentment with anger—partly because I've always had a hard time taking care of all the responsibilities that are mine and frequently need to find creative ways to take care of them. Which I do! Having to handle a whole new set of responsibilities was initially overwhelming.

Frankly, I wasn't aware of the many little and big things Carl routinely took care of until I've had to do them. For example, resetting the heating and air conditioners, handling the computer glitches that I regularly need help with, taking care of phone calls when I didn't want to be disturbed, buying the ingredients and preparing a meal, contacting professionals when we needed things repaired, keeping track of his own doctor and other appointments, and monitoring his medications. One of the hardest is that he no longer drives. This is a biggie, because he drove everywhere we wanted or needed to go and loved doing it. I drive well enough, but I hesitate to travel on superhighways or venture to places with which I'm not familiar. This is especially limiting, and I hate what it does to the freedom we used to have to take both long and short car trips. It also makes it necessary for us to respond with regrets to some invitations that we would like to accept. Our goddaughter and her parents are most willing to take us places, but that can get complicated. We don't feel comfortable asking people who invite us to include another guest, so we simply decline.

This is only a short list of the responsibilities that Carl used to take care of quietly and efficiently.

I still resist learning what I need to know to handle some of the technical stuff like the heating and air conditioning, and he still works with the system until he gets it adjusted. I know that soon I'll have to know what to do or get help, however.

Getting help is not a strategy that we yet have in place; however, we know that it is a practical way to ease the burden. Cost is a factor, and figuring that out is one of the steps we know we'll have to eventually take.

Although I know what is happening to Carl is not reversible and that it will progress, I keep what I describe as "healthy denial" in place. This somehow helps me to take the baby steps I need to take as new losses occur. And, surprisingly, I keep picking up where he leaves off without hardly noticing that I'm doing it.

Happily, my feelings of resentment are less than when I first had to do what he no longer could. What genuinely helps is that he is still aware of what is going on and is most appreciative. Interestingly, he smiles more than he used to, and we tend to laugh rather than get distressed at the foibles that catch us off guard.

The more that we both own, with grace, what is happening to him, the more we're able to say, "thanks" for what is still mostly good in each new day.

Q: What are some ways that I can remember that God is with and for both of us every minute of every day?

A: Throughout Carl's and my life together, the belief that God is with and for us always, has been deeply held. Yet, it surprises me that in the day-to-day challenges of the disease, I've wondered if I really believe that. And, in my self-talk I've sometimes pondered the probability of being naive regarding a God who supposedly loves and cares.

On the other hand, when I'm in the throes of self-doubt regarding my ability to hang in there, I find myself getting a second wind, a new surge of energy and strength. At those times, my faith reasserts itself, and my belief in a loving and supportive Other is affirmed.

An important thing that we do, and which I strongly recommend, as long as the person with Alzheimer's disease is able, is to go to church services. We happen to be blessed with liturgies that are lively song-filled celebrations with meaningful homilies that send us forth feeling challenged, refreshed, and strengthened. We had to search for this community. Luckily, we found one that nurtures and uplifts our spirit. It kind of sets the stage for each new week.

Another thing that I've found helpful is monitoring my self-talk. I'm talking to myself all the time, and gradually I'm learning to fine-tune what I'm saying so that, for example, self-pitying thoughts are quickly recognized and changed to thoughts about blessings; fearful and fretful thoughts are worked with and changed to "can do" ones; crippling thoughts about the future are changed to dealing with what has to be done right now, today. A good deal of my self-talk has focused

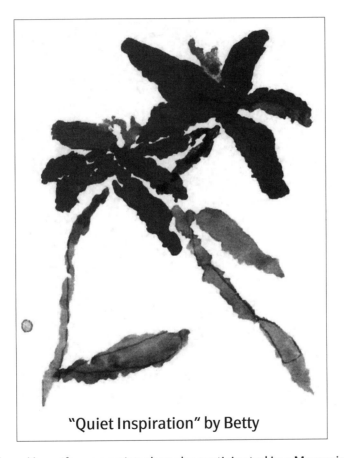

"Quiet Inspiration" by Betty

Betty found her gift as an artist when she participated in a Memories in the Making painting class. The art program pulls us into the inner world of an individual with Alzheimer's disease and allows a picture to communicate memories and experiences otherwise lost.

on the guilt I have about not being a good enough caregiver, a kind, loving and patient one. That becomes a refrain of forgiving myself and asking God to forgive, too. Frankly, I believe the latter is easier to come by than my own capacity to forgive.

And, still another thing that we have found genuinely helpful is having touchstones of our belief in every room of our home, like a crucifix or cross, a religious painting or statue, an open Bible on a stand in the entrance to our home, a piece of palm from Palm Sunday, and books of prayers like *The Blessing Cup* by Rock Travnikar, O.F.M. (St. Anthony Messenger Press, 1994) on our bookshelf, which we occasionally use for prayer.

Every family is different, so its religious practices and rituals will differ; however, chances are great that a response to "Is this all there is?" will be a recognition of Another helping us to make sense of what is going on and to know that in it there is more than what we can see and feel.

Having an opportunity to write this chapter is opening a new door for both of us. I have grown in my understanding of how we are with the disease, and he has been keenly interested and supportive. He even suggested that he is learning a lot about himself through it.

True Stories:
Relationships between Persons Affected by the Disease, Their Caregivers, Family Members, and Friends

Meet Connie Kudlacek, BS

Over the past 18 years, I have been the Executive Director of an Alzheimer's Association Chapter. During that time, I have been privileged to meet and work with many committed and dedicated individuals. These individuals were either actively caring for a loved one with dementia, volunteered or worked in a capacity of dealing with caregiving or geriatric issues, or had previously been a caregiver. Those who had been caregivers often devoted their time to helping others by sharing their experiences and contributing nonjudgmental advice to others who were experiencing the loss of their loved one to dementia. Previous to 1984, my husband and I were the primary caregivers to our oldest son, who sustained a traumatic brain injury at age 17 years and was left in need of total care.

What I have learned during all these years from families involved in crisis is how fragile we are as human beings and how each of us travels on a life journey equipped with certain coping skills and abilities. Sometimes, we caregivers give to another, even to the detriment of our own health.

I learned early in my role as caregiver for my son that others could take care of his daily needs, but only I could give him the love he needed from his mother. I was determined to stay healthy in mind, body, and spirit so that I could do that for him, and I often reached out to others to help me with this "caregiving of self."

My main focus with my son, with persons with dementia, and with all those who deal with the loss of their loved ones to dementia is first to recognize the dignity of persons and then to assist them with their needs.

As we become emotionally and physically exhausted from the demands of being a caregiver, we can lose sight of the essence of the person for whom we are caring, especially when an individual has dementia. We can become so involved in the daily tasks of taking physical care of our loved ones that we have little or no energy for nurturing the person within. My goal for this handbook is to offer caregivers tools that nurture them, that recognize their ability to make decisions that are in the best interests of all concerned. I feel that we all have certain coping skills, and we can learn new ones. This handbook is designed to enable caregivers to recognize their skills and meet their challenges with confidence in the choices they make.

Four other individuals have contributed to this handbook. Each part contributes to the overall message of concentrating on the "dignity within" the person with dementia and the caregiver. The tools and knowledge that the handbook give to you are our gifts to continue to nurture and sustain you as you travel through life's challenges.

I truly believe that nothing is more powerful in this world than the unwavering commitment and love one human can give to another. I have been privileged to personally experience that love in my own family, within the countless individuals who volunteer or work for the Alzheimer's Association, and within those who turn to the Alzheimer's Association for guidance.

The all-consuming responsibilities of caregiving for persons with Alzheimer's disease and related dementia produce complex and contradictory responses within families. "The reality is that family members have different ways of dealing with the stresses of caring," reports Thomas Kirk, former Alzheimer's Association Vice President. "It is beneficial for families to work through these challenges; otherwise the primary caregiver will have an increased chance of burnout as the individual's disease progresses. Families need to engage in more frequent communication and establish a plan for sharing caregiving responsibilities." This is difficult to do without some guidelines to help caregivers make the often emotionally charged decisions. Wouldn't it be helpful to know that with every decision you have only three choices or three ways to act?

To help you do this, the following stories are situations that have occurred during the past 20 years. I know that, as you read the stories, you will see yourself in many of these situations. The stories give you an opportunity to role-play. What you will learn is that there are simple ways for you to begin to control your journey on life's path of being a caregiver. But the stories are just one small part of this handbook. My belief is that each person who reads this handbook will find stories to which he or she can strongly relate and draw nourishment.

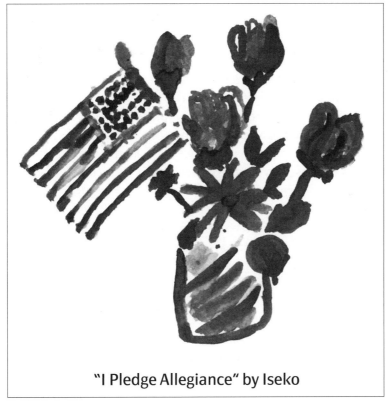

"I Pledge Allegiance" by Iseko

Iseko has been hard working all her life and was a skilled seamstress. She has always enjoyed painting, knitting, and making lovely Japanese floral arrangements. In the Memories in the Making program, we see stories of persons with Alzheimer's disease in a language that needs no words. Their paintings show us glimpses of who they were and who they still are.

Reading the Stories

On the following pages, you will find 20 stories describing the personal experiences of caregivers for individuals with dementia. Each story highlights one or two of the symptoms caregivers observed as they worked with persons with Alzheimer's disease or related dementia. We are grateful to the many people who were eager to share their perspectives and their journeys as caregivers.

As you read each story, pretend you are the caregiver in the situation. Think about the story and role-play what might happen within the context of your family situation. Present the situation to your personal "Advisory Board"—those favorite people from your past and present whose help you would like when important decisions need to be made (see Part I). They will suggest three different actions that you can take. The actions will be numbered 1, 2, or 3.

After reading each story, circle the response that best represents what you are most inclined to do. One response is not better than another, but may be more appropriate to use at certain times during the progression of Alzheimer's disease.

In addition, this handbook can help you do more than just role-play or reflect on caregiving situations. If you compile your responses on the "Summary Page" that follows, it can be used in Part IV to help you identify the style you most often use in your role as a caregiver. You will also learn about two alternative ways of acting if your "preferred style" does not allow you to stay positive in your role as caregiver. When you find yourself acting in a manner that removes dignity from your loved one or leaves you feeling like your own dignity has been lost, it may be time to:

- Take control;
- Let go of the situation; or
- Share responsibilities of caregiving with others.

SUMMARY PAGE

The "Summary Page" is provided for you to tabulate your caregiving style choices from the following 20 stories. Explanations of the three styles of caregiving will follow in Part IV of this handbook. You will be able to determine your "preferred style" as a caregiver and learn alternative styles to use as you continue to give care to persons with Alzheimer's disease or related dementia.

Check the number of the answer you indicated you would most likely do.

	1.	2.	3.
Situation # 1	_____	_____	_____
Situation # 2	_____	_____	_____
Situation # 3	_____	_____	_____
Situation # 4	_____	_____	_____
Situation # 5	_____	_____	_____
Situation # 6	_____	_____	_____
Situation # 7	_____	_____	_____
Situation # 8	_____	_____	_____
Situation # 9	_____	_____	_____
Situation #10	_____	_____	_____
Situation #11	_____	_____	_____
Situation #12	_____	_____	_____
Situation #13	_____	_____	_____
Situation #14	_____	_____	_____
Situation #15	_____	_____	_____
Situation #16	_____	_____	_____
Situation #17	_____	_____	_____
Situation #18	_____	_____	_____
Situation #19	_____	_____	_____
Situation #20	_____	_____	_____
TOTAL	_____	_____	_____
	YOU	WE	I

1. Why Can't Mother Remember?

Stage: Early-to-Mild Dementia

Symptoms: Decline in short term memory

Story: You and your sister take your mother out to dinner. You select one of your mother's favorite restaurants. Everyone is in good spirits and anticipates having a good time.

When you walk into the restaurant your mother says, "Oh, isn't this a lovely place! Look at the plates on the wall and the decorations. We will have to come here more often."

Your sister looks surprised and says, "Mom, you have been here a hundred times before. Don't you remember? We were just here last Easter, and . . ." You interrupt your sister and say, "Don't argue with her. Mom doesn't remember. Let's just sit down and have a nice dinner."

Because you spend more time with your mother than your sister does, you have experienced your mother's forgetfulness before. You know the times of forgetfulness are becoming more frequent.

CHALLENGE TO THE CAREGIVER:

How can you and your sister allow your mother to keep her dignity and independence and come to some agreement about mother's memory loss?

Styles of Primary Caregiver's Response:
In this situation, what might your next action be? (Circle one.)

1. You can ask your sister what she would be willing to do to better understand the situation. You can admit that you are struggling as a caregiver. You might say, "Is there any way you can help me out? I'm at my wits end." (YOU)
2. You and your sister can discuss the situation and decide that you both need to consult the family doctor and other experts to learn more about your mother's short and long-term prognosis. (WE)
3. You can take the lead and tell your sister what you have learned about your mother's symptoms. You can tell your sister about other incidents that have not gone well. You can say to your sister, "I plan to monitor mom's behavior and will stay on top of things. I'll be sure to keep you informed." (I)

My Thoughts/Notes:

_____

_____

_____

_____

When I was young, I could remember anything,
whether it happened or not.

—Mark Twain

2. How Can He Be So Insensitive?

Stage: Early-to-Mild Dementia
Symptoms: May be unreasonable and not realize it
Story: Your dad has lived alone in his house for many years and is now 95 years old. Two falls have put him in the hospital. After all the physical therapy allowed by insurance, the social worker and doctor tell you he needs around the clock care, and he cannot go back to his home alone. The doctor has diagnosed him with mild dementia and suggests that your dad can either go to a dementia-specific assisted living facility or you can arrange for around-the-clock care in his home.

You discuss the situation with your father. Financially and physically, around-the-clock care in the home is not possible. Your dad agrees to go to an assisted living facility.

The night before the move to the facility, you visit your dad. You are excited that you were able to arrange things the way he wants them. You say, "Dad, everything is ready for you. I think you are going to like it! I've arranged that you don't have to go down to breakfast if you don't want to ..." Dad cuts you off. "I'm not going! I only want to go home!" You remind your dad that he cannot live alone. "The doctor and social worker say you won't be safe alone at home." Dad says, "I'm not going." You respond with, "Yes, you are! They won't let you stay in the hospital any longer." You begin to argue back and forth.

CHALLENGE TO THE CAREGIVER:

How can you continue to provide for your father's needs without letting his reactions, due to the disease, hook you emotionally?

Style of Primary Caregiver's Response:
Which response would you most likely choose? (Circle one.)

1. Knowing that living alone is a dangerous situation for your dad and that getting irritated with him won't help things, you can carry through with the plans and simply end the conversation by saying, "We will see, Dad." (YOU)
2. You could call Dad's friends and his doctor and ask them to explain the situation to your father and help him adjust to this move. (WE)
3. You could leave, get some distance, and talk with someone about the situation. You can try to appreciate your dad's difficulty in adapting to this big change in his lifestyle. You can remind yourself that his apparent insensitivity to your needs is part of the early stages of dementia and try not to take his comments personally. (I)

MY THOUGHTS/NOTES:

_____

_____

_____

_____

The whole worth of a kind deed lies in the love that inspires it.
—The Talmud

3. Is This the Person I Married?

Stage: Early-to-Mild Dementia
Symptoms: More withdrawn; less socially interactive; less outgoing
Story: You are a prominent lawyer and your wife has been diagnosed with early stage Alzheimer's disease. You are both well known in the community for your good works and the prominence of your children. You frequently attend community functions and work on issues of social justice.

You and your wife are attending a party where many people know you. In the conversation, your wife is asked some questions. She appears confused and doesn't know what to answer. You answer for her to keep the conversation going. When this happens, your wife seems embarrassed and becomes agitated. You are also embarrassed.

Incidents like this are becoming more frequent. The anger and frustration you both are experiencing is becoming obvious to your children. No one seems to be doing anything about the situation, and things are become more tense within the family.

CHALLENGE TO THE CAREGIVER:

As the husband, how can you honor where your wife is as she copes with Alzheimer's disease and yet help to alleviate situations that cause embarrassment and anger that impacts the entire family?

Styles of Primary Caregiver's Response:
In this situation, what might your next action be? (Circle one.)

1. You can speak privately with your wife and encourage her to seek medical help to understand her behavioral changes and then work with her on establishing new interpersonal arrangements that will be comfortable for both of you. (YOU)
2. You and your children can be patient and wait for your wife to seek professional counseling. Once she seeks help, you all can make plans to accommodate her changing needs then adjust your lifestyles to support her in her decisions. (WE)
3. You and the children, along with concerned friends, can conduct an intervention with your wife to force the issue and begin the process of dialogue. (I)

MY THOUGHTS/NOTES:

_____

_____

_____

_____

Almost all our faults are more pardonable
than the methods we think up to hide them.
                    —La Rochefoucauld

4. Is It Okay If I Don't Tell the Truth?

Stage: Early-to-Mild Dementia

Symptoms: Forgets things that happened; can say insensitive things

Story: It is Christmas time. You and your sister Anne are going shopping. You have money to spend, but Anne is on a limited budget. Your mother, who has early signs of dementia, gives Anne $300 to do her shopping and tells her to use the rest to shop for her family.

When you return home after shopping, you both show your mother all the things you bought. You are having a great time—laughing and showing excitement like children yourselves. Out of the blue, your mother asks Anne, "Why did you buy so much? You don't earn that much money. No wonder you are always broke." Your mother has forgotten that she gave Anne the money.

While knowing your mother has early dementia, neither of you are ready to cope with this aspect of the disease. You are both confused, hurt, and sad and don't quite know how to respond. You want to rescue your sister and say, "Mom, what do you mean? You gave Anne the money. She isn't to blame." But you remember another time when you came to Anne's defense and, at that time, your mother replied, "I did not! You are making that up!"

CHALLENGE TO THE CAREGIVER:

How do you and your sister cope with the hurt feelings you experience as you watch your mother's memory diminish?

Styles of Primary Caregiver's Response:
In this situation, what might your next action be? (Circle one.)

1. You and your sister can acknowledge that your mother's behavior is part of the disease. You can agree, when this happens again, you will try to defuse the emotion by using humor. You might agree to say, "We won the lottery—don't worry about the money, Mom." (YOU)

2. You and your sister can agree to document incidents indicating the dates, times, and events of any disturbing behavior patterns your mother exhibits and share this information with your mother's doc-

tor. You may also agree to get some personal counseling to deal with the anger, hurt, and guilt you may be feeling. (WE)

3. You and your sister can agree to educate yourselves on the progression of Alzheimer's disease to learn what is happening in your Mom's brain to cause her to say insensitive things. Once you have the facts, it may be easier to deal with the strong emotions you are feeling. (I)

MY THOUGHTS/NOTES:

_____

_____

_____

_____

*I don't believe life is supposed to make you feel
good, or to make you feel miserable either.
Life is just supposed to make you feel.*
—Gloria Naylor

5. How Should We Handle the News That It's Dementia?

Stage: Early-to-Mild Dementia
Symptoms: Confusion; social withdrawal
Story: Your wife, Karen, is 58 years old and works as a mail carrier. She complains that she is sometimes confused while driving her route. She places mail for one address into another resident's box. At first, she attributed this "forgetfulness" to personal stress. You are beginning to notice Karen's forgetfulness too. She seems to be withdrawing from social interactions with friends and family.

In discussion, Karen admits to you that she misplaces items of everyday use and then is unable to remember that she has even handled them. She says when your daughters come with their families, she just wants to be in her room and doesn't feel like socializing.

Concerned, you seek help from a geriatric assessment center. The diagnosis is early stage dementia with some mild depression. The geriatric physician recommends that Karen begin taking a new medication for Alzheimer's disease.

You are anticipating how both of your lives might change. Her early retirement would mean a major reduction in your income, because you are already on disability due to a work-related injury. You often become angry and impatient with Karen's forgetfulness and withdrawal. You have told your children that they cannot all come at the same time to visit and need to stay for shorter periods. Your daughters do not accept that their mother has Alzheimer's disease and often blame you for some of her behaviors and for not being supportive and more understanding of her.

CHALLENGE TO THE CAREGIVER:

How do you balance the need for a primary wage earner with your wife's increasing demands for emotional and physical help?

Styles of Primary Caregiver's Response:
In this situation, what might your next action be? (Circle one.)

1. You can continue to monitor Karen's behavior, noting favorable and unfavorable changes that occur. You can be supportive of her retirement and assure her that you will find ways for her to contribute to the household. (YOU)
2. You and Karen can have a family meeting with all the children and a medical person who will educate all of you concerning the possible long-term affects of dementia. Family members can be challenged to become involved in any long-term financial adjustments the family might have to make. (WE)
3. You can continue to educate yourself on the effects of Alzheimer's disease and hope that the medicine will bring Karen back to a more healthy way of acting. You can get yourself psychologically and emotionally ready for the caregiving that will follow by putting into place a personal support system. (I)

MY THOUGHTS/NOTES:

_____

_____

_____

_____

Whatever you are be a good one.
—Abraham Lincoln

6. How Do I Know If Something Is Wrong?

Stage: Early-to-Mild Dementia
Symptoms: Withdrawn; forgetful
Story: I've been a certified public accountant for 25 years and just turned 59 this past summer. I was working for a prominent firm, but was recently discharged from my position. The firm said I made numerous errors over the past two years, which resulted in lost business for them. They did discuss these errors with me, and I thought I reassured them that I was fully capable of doing my job. Nonetheless, they dismissed me saying that I was a liability for their firm. My wife has recently noticed that I am more forgetful. She tells me I seem more withdrawn.

She says it could be the stress over losing my job or the fact that I will soon be 60 years old. In any case, I am angry because I was dismissed and because I don't feel there's anything wrong. I do know I could easily get depressed if I have to sit around the house all day and can't work.

CHALLENGE TO THE CAREGIVER:

How do you and your wife face your diminishing capacity and still view your life as productive?

Styles of Primary Caregiver's Response:
In this situation, what might your next action be? (Circle one.)

1. You can refuse to seek help. Your wife may be forced to confront you more directly about how your behavior is impacting your life together. She can make demands and set out conditions and insist that you follow them. (YOU)
2. You and your wife can agree to monitor your behavior more closely, documenting activities that indicate the possible presence of dementia. You can agree that, at a certain point, you will get a geriatric assessment or seek help from an objective third party if conditions do not improve. (WE)
3. Because you are your own caregiver, you can consult a specialist to talk about the angry feelings you are experiencing. This consultation, in dealing with emotions, could lead you to seek further care for your physical well-being. (I)

MY THOUGHTS/NOTES:

_____

_____

_____

_____

The best educated human being is the one who
understands most about the life in which he is placed.
—Helen Keller

7. Would My Mother Become Violent with Her Own Sister?

Stage: Early-to-Mild Dementia
Symptoms: Trouble naming things and finding the right words; arguing and frustration, because people do not understand
Story: You are a single parent and head of the household for your mother, age 76, and your son, age 14.

In addition, you recently brought your aunt, age 81, into your home because she was diagnosed with dementia and has difficulty naming things and expressing herself.

One day, when you return home from work, you see your mother and aunt arguing. Your mother keeps correcting your aunt whenever she gives a wrong answer to your mother's question. Your mother does not appear to relate this behavior to a disease. Out of frustration, your mother raises her hand as if to strike your aunt, but then refrains from doing so.

You observe the possibility of your mother becoming physically violent toward your aunt. You know your mother doesn't mean to be impatient, but perhaps the frustration of dealing with your aunt's dementia is too great for your mom.

CHALLENGE TO THE CAREGIVER:

How do you help your mother realize that your aunt's actions are caused by a disease and are not intentional?

Styles of Primary Caregiver's Response:
In this situation, what might your next action be? (Circle one.)

1. You can coach your mother through the difficult times, assuring her that what she is experiencing with her sister is because of her sister's changing behavior. However, as a caregiver, your mother will need to be aware of her own emotional and physical needs and get some distance from the caregiving process. (YOU)
2. You and your mom can attend an Alzheimer's support group to learn more about the caregiver's role and how the continued progression of Alzheimer's disease will impact the family. You can work together and arrange times when home health care can attend to your aunt while you are away at work. (WE)
3. You can schedule times when you will care for your aunt so that your mother can take time away and regain her emotional control and/or learn more about the effects of the disease and what is happening in the brain. (I)

MY THOUGHTS/NOTES:

_____

_____

_____

_____

Lord, give me the wisdom to make
stepping stones out of stumbling blocks.
                              —Anonymous

8. Who Has Power of Attorney?

Stage: Early-to-Mild Dementia
Symptoms: Forgetfulness
Story: You and Pearl have been married for six years. You are now in your early 70s, and this is a second marriage for both of you. When Pearl's husband died, you contacted her to renew your high school friendship. Pearl has two sons, and they were fine with the marriage because they felt Pearl would have difficulty living alone and managing her property. The boys live in other parts of the country and do not visit often—although they communicate with you and their mother frequently by phone and e-mail.

Over the past 18 months, Pearl has become totally dependent on you. She had always shown signs of forgetfulness, so you began managing her financial affairs along with planning all daily activities since the start of the marriage. You also took Pearl to her family physician, who told her she suffered from some form of dementia. After a complete geriatric assessment, the doctors recommended that Pearl participate in a drug trial study to see if a new dementia-specific drug might help her.

In previous studies, this drug was shown to have some possible severe side effects. Because of this, Pearl's sons feel that she should not take part in the study. You have Power of Attorney for both health and finances. You want to respect the sons' position but also want to do all you can to help Pearl.

CHALLENGE TO THE CAREGIVER:

How do you convince your new sons that you are interested in Pearl's best welfare and maintain the even stronger family relationship which is needed now?

Styles of Primary Caregiver's Response:
In this situation, what might your next action be? (Circle one.)

1. You can contact the sons and share with them information about Pearl's condition. You will have to tell them that, if she does not participate in this drug study, she may need to be medicated to calm her reactions to daily events. You can ask them to make the final decision about Pearl's participation in the trial drug and tell them you will abide by their decision. (YOU)

2. Even though you have Power of Attorney, you can ask the sons to talk with Pearl's doctor. Then, together, you, the sons, and the doctor can decide the best course of action for Pearl. (WE)

3. You can contact the sons and share with them information about Pearl's condition, behavior, and assessment. You can tell them the alternatives in her long-term care that might be necessary. You can outline the pros and cons of taking or not taking the new trial drug. Through dialogue, you can try to convince the sons that you will do everything in Pearl's best interest, but ultimately you will make the final decision. (I)

My Thoughts/Notes:

_____

_____

_____

_____

The greatest thing you can do for another is not
just to share your riches, but to reveal to him his own.
—Benjamin Disraeli

9. Whose Rights Prevail?

Stage: Early-to-Mild Dementia, related to Parkinson's disease and Lewy body dementia
Symptoms: Motor problems of Parkinson's disease (tremors, freezing, unsteadiness); forgetfulness
Story: After your mom died, your dad, who has Parkinson's disease, began living with your brother. Your dad does not have sufficient finances to live alone and care for himself. Your brother has to work many hours to earn a living. By living together, they are able to share expenses and maintain their house. When your brother is home, he and your dad like to smoke while watching TV. Your dad has been a smoker all of his adult life.

You are the only daughter in the family and live in Florida with your own family. You work full time and are unable to take care of your father, but you are very concerned about his living conditions.

As your dad's Parkinson's disease has progressed, he often has uncontrollable tremors. The doctor has prescribed medication, but he forgets to take it. Many days, he is unable to get out of bed or the lounge chair in which he falls asleep. When you call, he gets mad at your questions and screams at you over the phone. You have grave concerns about your dad being left alone so much because of the progression of his Parkinson's. You worry when he smokes. You have discussed this with your brother, who simply says he won't stop your dad from smoking because it is their way of relaxing together.

Because of your brother's financial constraints, you know dad and your brother are not able to hire daily assistance for your dad's care.

You cannot move your dad in with you because of your own commitment to your job and family and lack of space within your home.

CHALLENGE TO THE CAREGIVER:

How do you and your brother provide for your dad's current needs while encouraging him to be responsible for his behaviors?

Styles of Primary Caregiver's Response:
In this situation, what might your next action be? (Circle one.)

1. Understanding the fact that your dad and brother will probably keep smoking, you could purchase a flame resistant apron from a home health store for your father to wear. You can also negotiate with your brother to restrict smoking to only certain areas of the home. (YOU)
2. You and your brother could seek assistance from the Area Agency on Aging's in-home assistance program, and you could contribute financially to hire additional assistance where needed. (WE)
3. You could move your dad to Florida and place him in a nursing home. (I)

MY THOUGHTS/NOTES:

_____

_____

_____

_____

Keep your fears to yourself, but share your courage.
—Robert Louis Stevenson

10. Where Are the Keys?

Stage: Moderate Dementia
Symptoms: Loses things; gets confused
Story: Your mother, who has been diagnosed with Alzheimer's disease, lives alone and shows signs that this may not be a good arrange-

ment for very much longer. She still drives, but she has driven the car, left it in a parking lot, and "someone" had to bring her home. She did not remember where she left the car. She wants to manage her life and financial affairs, but you learn that she has not been paying her bills.

You have been given Power of Attorney for your mother's day-to-day responsibilities. Your sisters, who live in different parts of the country, do not think there is much wrong with Mother. When they talk with her on the phone, she seems delightful and just fine. Mother tells your sisters that you are mean to her and that you take the car keys away. Because of this situation, you do not have the support of your sisters to make the necessary decisions that are required to keep your mom safe.

Your mother has substantial financial resources, and you believe that if she is in a car accident the family would be sued and this might leave no financial resources for your mother's continued care.

CHALLENGE TO THE CAREGIVER:

How do you continue to be the primary caregiver, knowing other members of the family will not support your decisions?

Styles of Primary Caregiver's Response:
In this situation, what might your next action be? (Circle one.)

1. Understanding the family dynamics, you could continue interacting with your mother as best you can. You can let your mother drive the car, and the next time she forgets where it is, you could have it towed away and impounded. You might also suggest to your sisters that Mother come and visit with them for a week or two, so that they can see first hand how she is coping with daily events. (YOU)
2. You could call a meeting of your sisters to discuss the family situation and ask if someone else would like to be given Power of Attorney, since they are unhappy with the decisions you are making. (WE)
3. You could tell your sisters that, while you are designated the person with Power of Attorney, even if they are not in full agreement with your decisions, you must first be concerned about Mother's safety needs. (I)

MY THOUGHTS/NOTES:

_____

_____

_____

_____

Give others a piece of your heart,
not a piece of your mind.
> —Anonymous

11. Who Comes First?

Stage: Moderate Dementia

Symptoms: Inability to function independently; difficulty with problem solving

Story: Your sister Jeanne, who lives in Seattle, arrives in Omaha to help you review the care of your mother. You have three young children and have been taking care of your mother for over a year, but you can no longer manage your mother's care and the needs of your family.

You soon discover that Jeanne has high expectations of care for Mother. Jeanne regrets that she does not live closer to you to help with the responsibilities. The fact that your mother is only 68 and can no longer live independently is troublesome to both of you. You see that she has been having greater difficulty with managing her finances and cooking, and she sometimes gets lost when by herself. You believe your mother will live quite a long life. The energy and finances to give continuous high-quality care is of great concern to both of you.

As you continue to work together, you realize you cannot keep up with Jeanne's expectations. The relationship between the two of you is becoming strained.

CHALLENGE TO THE CAREGIVER:

How do you and your sister provide for the long-term care of your Mother and also take care of some of your own personal needs?

Styles of Primary Caregiver's Response:
In this situation, what might your next action be? (Circle one.)

1. You, Jeanne, and your mother can discuss your mother's wishes in terms of long-term care. You can agree to fulfill her wishes to the best of your ability. You can also agree to call in an arbitrary third party to make the objective decisions that may be too difficult for you to make. (YOU)
2. You, Jeanne, and your mother can seek out early support groups where newly diagnosed persons with Alzheimer's disease can speak freely with others in a similar situation. You can all ask questions and gain additional information about practical issues to help you make the long-term decisions that will lie ahead. With this new knowledge, you and your sister can decide who would be best to take the lead at different times in the caregiving process. (WE)
3. You and Jeanne can make a plan for long-term continued care, after gaining information about assisted living facilities, financial assessments, and other health care options. You can take the responsibility to make certain the care plan is followed. (I)

MY THOUGHTS/NOTES:

_____

_____

_____

_____

*You gain strength, courage, and confidence by every
experience which you must stop and look fear in the face...
you must do the thing you think you cannot do.*
                                        —Eleanor Roosevelt

12. Who Does the Changing?

Stage: Moderate Dementia
Symptoms: Paranoid
Story: Your mom and dad have been in an assisted living facility for four years. At first, they took part in some of the activities, but now they have become withdrawn, often hostile to the residents, and accuse other residents of stealing things. When other relatives visit your parents, they do not see this type of disturbing behavior. They tell you that

your parents are just getting older, and behavior changes are to be expected.

But when you go to see them, they often seem confused and dwell on events from the past. They become angry with you and accuse you of wanting to put them in a nursing home so you can get their money. You leave each visit feeling angry with your parents. You don't like the way your relationship with them is changing. You think your parents are really angry with the situation and their inability to do things which were once easy for them.

CHALLENGE TO THE CAREGIVER:

How do you cope with your own anger and still keep personal contact with your parents?

Styles of Primary Caregiver's Response:
In this situation, what might your next action be? (Circle one.)

1. You can resign yourself to the fact that your mother and father may continue to act this way. Because of your strong feelings you may decide it is best to just visit with them over the phone rather than visit in person. (YOU)
2. You can think about taking your parents places where they can enjoy the socialization and try to get them out more when you visit or bring a friend with you when you visit. (WE)
3. You can speak with the officials of the assisted living facility about your observations. You can request a review of their medication with the doctor. You may decide to continue seeing them, but not as often, and only go when you are emotionally strong. (I)

MY THOUGHTS/NOTES:

_____

_____

_____

_____

When we are well, we all have good advice for those who are ill.
—Lucius Annaeus Seneca

13. How Was I to Know?

Stage: Moderate Dementia
Symptoms: Self-care problems; disorientation
Story: Your dad, Henry, until his sudden death, was a loving husband to your mother, Belle. As an adopted son, you travel to the homestead in Kentucky for the funeral. You have not seen your parents for a number of years, because your dad always reported that everything was all right. At the funeral home, while making arrangements for your father, you discover that he kept it a secret that your mom was showing the effects of dementia. You find your mother with some neighbors and relatives who have just discovered that your mother cannot understand what others are saying and cannot speak for what she needs.

Aunt Jane says, "Henry, I'm sorry to tell you, but I don't think your mom knows what's going on. She seems disoriented and asks the same questions over and over. We haven't seen your mom and dad for a long time . . . things come up. . . . You know how it is. . . . You're going to have to do something for your mom. She cannot be left alone."

You realize that your father used distance and travel expenses as reasons to discourage you from visiting. There was no way for you to know before now about your mother's condition. Your job and home are across the country. You need to make some immediate arrangements for your mother's safety and care.

CHALLENGE TO THE CAREGIVER:

How can you responsibly care for your mother and adjust to the news that she has dementia in such a short period of time?

Styles of Primary Caregiver's Response:
In this situation, what might your next action be? (Circle one.)

1. You can wait until your mother becomes less stressed and talk with her to discover what her wishes for continued care might be. (YOU)
2. You can talk with your wife, relatives, and the neighbors and together decide what the best course of action will be. You and your wife can offer to bring Mom to your home. (WE)
3. You can plan to stay with your mother and arrange for her to have a medical examination. You could coordinate a schedule with friends and neighbors to ensure that people check in on her several times a day until a more permanent solution can be found. (I)

My Thoughts/Notes:

_____

_____

_____

_____

Worry never robs tomorrow of its sorrows;
it only saps today of its strength.

—A. J. Cronin

14. Is There Caregiver Abuse?

Stage: Moderate Dementia
Symptoms: Anger; wandering; confusion
Story: Your parents live in a small rural town in the Midwest. They have lived there since leaving the farm two years ago, but have not made many acquaintances in town. They have been married for over 40 years and you are their only daughter. You live in another town.

Your father was diagnosed with Alzheimer's disease several years ago and has shown progressive signs of deterioration, leaving your mother to care for most of his needs. She has promised him that she would take care of him in their home and never put him in a nursing home.

Your father is not sleeping nights and wanders throughout the house, often calling for your mother. He becomes agitated when she is out of his sight, yet when she tries to assist him with dressing or bathing, he yells at her. There are no adult day care programs or formal in-home services in the rural area where they live. Your mother is taking care of your father night and day by herself, draining her own physical and emotional energy.

When you come for your usual bimonthly visit, you notice Dad's arms. When you ask your mother about them, she explains that your father was unsure of his balance and fell several times. She seems less willing to discuss your father's care with you, and she even discourages you from visiting.

CHALLENGE TO THE CAREGIVER:

The primary caregiver is now in need of a caregiver to gain perspective on issues. As their daughter, how do you help your mom recognize that she is no longer able to handle her own emotions while dealing with your dad's condition?

Styles of Primary Caregiver's Response:
In this situation, what would your next action be? (Circle one.)

1. If your mother is open to the idea of counseling, you can encourage her to seek this help to gain some emotional relief. (YOU)
2. You and your mother can hire assistance to come in daily to take care of your dad in his home. This will give relief to your mother and help her gain a healthy perspective so that she can continue to care for her husband. (WE)
3. You can explore options with the Area Agency on Aging Case Manager Division to get information on the state's requirements for application for Spousal Impoverishment prior to placing your father in a nursing home. This law protects spouses from losing all their assets to pay for their partner's care. When you take the lead in finding a nursing home, your mother can still keep her promise that she would never place her husband in a home. (I)

MY THOUGHTS/NOTES:

_____

_____

_____

_____

It is not doing the thing we like to do, but liking
the thing we have to do, that makes life blessed.
                                        —Goethe

15. Should a Caregiver Be On Call 24/7?

Stage: Moderate-to-Severe Dementia
Symptoms: Sleep disturbances; behavior and personality changes
Story: Your mom has Alzheimer's disease, and the disease is progressing. Your father was taking care of your mother until your mother started wandering at night. When this happened, your father couldn't get to sleep and became ill himself. You and your dad looked for a suitable place for your mother to go. You moved her into an assisted living facility, but found it did not meet your mother's care needs.

You then moved her into a dementia-specific assisted living facility. The staff at the assisted living facility cannot supervise her 24 hours a day. She is wandering into other residents' rooms and exhibiting some unacceptable behaviors. You do not want to move her again.

Your dad says he will try to take care of her at home one more time, but you do not want to jeopardize your father's health. You work full-time and cannot stop working to take care of your mother.

CHALLENGE TO THE CAREGIVER:

How do you balance your need to stay healthy and assist your father in the care of your mother?

Styles of Primary Caregiver's Response:
In this situation, what might your next action be? (Circle one.)

1. You and your father, knowing the assisted living facility is the best place for your mother, can decide to leave her there but work with the facility to help with her adjustment. (YOU)
2. You and your father can agree to allow your mother to return home under certain conditions. Those conditions are that home health care be brought in to assist with your mother's physical needs and time be set aside for your father to take daily respite. (WE)
3. You and your father can agree to allow your father to care for your mother one more time, under certain conditions. When caregiving begins to affect your father's health again, you will become the primary caregiver and no longer depend on joint decisions with your father. (I)

My Thoughts/Notes:

_____

_____

_____

_____

I believe in the Sun ... when it is not shining;
I believe in Love... even when I feel it not;
I believe in God ... even when He is silent.
                              —Irish Blessing/Proverb

16. Should We Use Restraints or Medication—
What Is the Priority?

Stage: Moderate-to-Severe Dementia
Symptoms: Hallucinations; safety issues
Story: For the past six years you have been regularly visiting your dad, Ernie, who lives in a nursing home. You have two other sisters who also take turns visiting him. Your dad has difficulty finding the appropriate words for objects and does not always recognize his family. Sometimes he mixes his children's and grandchildren's names.

Your dad often shows extreme agitation, and he hallucinates. He often wanders within the unit day and night. He has begun to fall frequently. Recently, he broke his arm and his nose. Your family insists that the staff at the facility restrain him so that he does not fall and hurt himself. Your family has been informed by the facility that state law will not allow them to restrain your dad even for his own protection. However, he could be placed on a medication that may make him more sedate. You do not want your dad sedated to the point where he is unresponsive and immobile.

Challenge to the Caregiver:

How does Ernie's family, who are not his direct caregivers, provide for his safety when he is living in a nursing home?

Styles of Primary Caregiver's Response:
In this situation, what would your next action be? (Circle one)

1. You and your sisters could work with the staff to get the appropriate level of medication to calm your dad. This would allow the staff to work with him more appropriately. (YOU)
2. You and your sisters could work with the staff at the current facility to develop a care plan that would include your participation in monitoring his activities. (WE)
3. You could contact the doctor for a further medical examination and request that orders be written for a type of restraint that would provide for your dad's safety needs. (I)

MY THOUGHTS/NOTES:

_____

_____

_____

_____

Roads are meant for journeys not destinations.
—Anonymous

17. How Do I Know It's Not Just Old Age?

Stage: Moderate-to-Severe Dementia
Symptoms: Hallucinations; self-care problems; safety issues; incoherent
Story: Maria, who is 80 years old, lives with you and your husband in a metropolitan city in the United States. You and your husband immigrated from Mexico and have been living and working in the city for the past four years. As soon as Maria came to live with you, you realized that she was having memory problems and was sometimes confused. You remembered that before she came to the United States, she sometimes wandered from her village in Mexico.

To financially sustain the family you and your husband must work, often 12 hours a day. Maria is left alone for extended periods. She watches television or sleeps. Sometimes she hallucinates about the stories on television and becomes frightened. If she sees her reflection in a mirror she will scream and strike out at it. At times she babbles incoherently and has begun to soil herself. When you and your husband come home from work, Maria hides from you or tries to escape from the home.

In your culture, you were taught to believe that Maria's behavior is just a symptom of old age. You feel that it is necessary to lock her in the house when you leave for work for two reasons. One is for her own safety and to prevent her from wandering away, but the second is also serious. Maria has entered the country illegally and you are fearful that if the authorities find out she is living with you, she will be returned to Mexico.

Challenge to the Caregiver:

How do you change your view of Maria's behavior and recognize her behavior is more than just a symptom of old age? How do you develop a plan that will meet her physical and emotional needs?

Styles of Primary Caregiver's Response:
In this situation, what might your next action be? (Circle one.)

1. Because culturally Maria's condition is viewed as a symptom of old age, you and your husband may continue to lock her in the house. When and if Maria does something that is harmful to herself, others, or things, you may be forced to take more direct action. (YOU)
2. You and your husband could talk to your priest or minister about the situation. The priest/minister could put you in contact with the Alzheimer's chapter for resources. (WE)
3. Caregivers have a responsibility to seek help and become informed about the needs of their loved one. You and your husband can take Maria for a physical examination at a health clinic in the Hispanic community and learn from professionals what would be a safe course of action for Maria. (I)

My Thoughts/Notes:

_____

_____

_____

_____

One isn't necessarily born with courage,
but one is born with potential. Without courage,
we cannot practice any other virtue with consistency.
We can't be kind, true, merciful, generous, or honest.
                                    —Maya Angelou

18. Who Needs Help The Caregiver or the Person With Dementia?

Stage: Severe Dementia
Symptoms: Safety and self-care issues arise; hallucinations
Story: You have two more years before you can take early retirement. You are behind in your work and are concerned about losing your job. You are also experiencing some medical problems with high blood pressure. You worry and care for your wife, Sonja, who is in her early 60s and has Alzheimer's disease.

Sonja has been attending an adult day care program during weekdays for the past two years. In the morning, Sonja is often aggressive towards you—striking out when you try to assist her in dressing. Each morning, it is a battle getting her up, fed, and dressed to go to the day care program. Once she is there, she enjoys the social interaction with the other residents.

Recently, Sonja has begun to hide items. At home, she hallucinates about situations she sees on the television and imagines that they are actually happening. Last evening, Sonja wandered away from you while you were out shopping and got into a stranger's car.

CHALLENGE TO THE CAREGIVER:

How can you care for your wife, who has advanced care needs, and still work to produce needed income?

Styles of Primary Caregiver's Response:
In this situation, what might your next action be? (Circle one.)

1. Because Sonja cannot be responsible for her daily care, you can seek medical assistance and have Sonja evaluated for possible drug therapy that can help to calm her. (YOU)
2. If finances are not available, you can seek legal counsel and request special resource allowances under the Medicare Catastrophic

Coverage Act of 1988. This federal law protects spouses from losing all their assets to pay for a partner's care. (Laws pertaining to this act differ from state to state.) (WE)

3. If finances are available, you can place Sonja in a nursing home, admitting that both your physical welfare are at stake in this situation. (I)

My Thoughts/Notes:

_____

_____

_____

_____

The journey of a thousand miles begins with a single step.
—Lao Tse

19. Can You Accept Me For Who I Am Today?

Stage: Severe Dementia
Symptoms: Incontinent and immobile
Story: You frequently visit your mother in a nursing home and always check with personnel about changes in your mother's condition. Your mother is mostly immobile, incontinent, and has difficulty swallowing. For the last month or so, your mother has not recognized you, but talks with you as if you were someone else.

Today, when you visit, you greet your mother, who is sitting in a wheelchair. Again, your mother looks at you but does not seem to recognize you. You tell her that you are her daughter Janice. Your mother calls you Emily and asks about her brother Frank. You realize Emily was your grandmother. You try to tell your mother that Frank and Emily died many years ago. But your mother mumbles something that you do not understand. Your mother becomes restless and agitated.

You know your mom is incapable of self-care and has severe memory loss, but you are hurt by the fact that she could not recognize you.

CHALLENGE TO THE CAREGIVER:

How do you balance the losses you are experiencing with your mother and be mindful of the dignity that remains throughout the disease process?

Styles of Primary Caregiver's Response:
In this situation, what might your next action be? (Circle one)

1. You could just relax and let your mother continue with her own thoughts and be present to your mother by listening quietly. (YOU)
2. You could enter into a dialogue with your mother and pretend to be Emily and reminisce along with your mom. (WE)
3. You can continue to try and get your mother to recognize you. You may never accomplish this, however, and frustration and arguments may occur. (I)

MY THOUGHTS/NOTES:

_____

_____

_____

_____

When someone you love becomes a memory,
the memory becomes a treasure.
　　　　　—Trudy Newman, Past Caregiver

20. To Hold On or Let Go?

Stage: Severe Dementia, related to Pick's disease
Symptoms: Total care needs; nutritional problems
Story: Over the past four years, your husband, Tyrone, who has Pick's disease, has lived in a nursing home. Previously, Tyrone was an active person who regularly spent time with you, his children, and grandchildren. You visit the nursing home daily and feed Tyrone lunch. On occasion, Tyrone will appear to recognize you. Many other family members visit, often sharing memories and stories of the past.

Tyrone is now bedridden, incontinent, and not able to swallow appropriately. At this time, Tyrone requires total care. The physician at the facility where Tyrone resides has informed you that he is not taking nutrition and has suggested that a feeding tube be inserted to assist with appropriate nutrition and hydration.

You want to have this procedure done because you do not want him to starve to death. Tyrone's adult children are concerned about prolonging his life because they see his quality of life as unbearable for him. The doctor has informed the family that a person does not experience discomfort if the dying process is allowed to take place naturally. As long as he recognizes you, you do not want to give up hope. A decision needs to be made.

CHALLENGE TO THE CAREGIVER:

How does Tyrone's family resolve their differences and accept end-of-life issues?

Styles of Primary Caregiver's Response:
In this situation, what might your next action be? (Circle one.)

1. Believing that Tyrone would not want extraordinary means to prolong his life, the family could keep their father comfortable and pain free and allow the dying process to take its course. (YOU)
2. The family could get another opinion, which would mean starting over with another doctor. They would buy some time before an ultimate decision would have to be made about the insertion of a feeding tube to extend their father's life. (WE)
3. Unable or unwilling to let the father die, the family can prolong life by asking the doctor to insert the feeding tube. (I)

MY THOUGHTS/NOTES:

_____

_____

_____

_____

Lord, give me eyes that I may see lest I, as people will,
should pass by someone's Calvary and think it is just a hill.
                                        —Anonymous

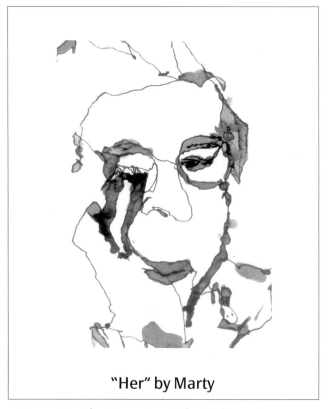

"Her" by Marty

In creating the Memories in the Making art program, the Alzheimer's team employed many techniques to find what evoked interest in their patients. When doing contour drawings, they were instructed to draw looking only at the subject and not at their pens or pencils. This directive can frustrate many art students, but it didn't faze Marty. She just went ahead and drew "Her" (the instructor) without a pause.

IV

Caregiving Styles: Three Ways to Respond

Meet Barbara C. Vasiloff, MA

My life as a caregiver has been primarily to students. Although it is true that students have many social, emotional, and intellectual needs, as a teacher I have not yet cared for a person with Alzheimer's disease or other dementia.

My parents have been blessed with good health and longevity and, while my 87-year-old mother shows some signs of forgetfulness, no one in our family would suggest that she has early Alzheimer's disease .

My family believes mental and physical health has much to do with attitude and perspective. We believe that, when mom's symptoms become self-evident, we will be ready to face these facts and deal with a different kind of caregiving. For now, my father, who is 89, is a loving, constant companion who assists, coaches, argues, reshapes mom's thinking to fit ongoing realities, and allows himself these same interactions from my mother.

Therefore, my contribution to this handbook is somewhat different from Pat's, Roger's, Janaan's, and Connie's. I have been an educator for over 30 years and am currently a Lecturer in the Department of

Education in the College of Arts and Sciences at Creighton University. I am co-founder of Discipline with Purpose, Inc., which offers a developmental approach to teaching self-discipline. Our organization specializes in teaching 15 self-discipline skills to educators, parents and students.

Many of the self-discipline skills are critical to effective caregiving. The ability to listen, communicate, resolve problems, initiate solutions, distinguish fact from feeling, and be of service to others are essential skills a caregiver must learn to perform. As an educator, I offer the caregivers an organized way to recognize the options open to them when making decisions.

Making good decisions requires self-discipline. Self-discipline is a person's ability to wait and, while waiting, to think about how to act. Usually, this is done so instantaneously that the separate components that lead toward the eventual action are not considered. When we do reflect on these components, we realize that there are three patterns or styles used by most decision-makers. These styles take into consideration the amount of power and/or control the decision-maker will keep or give away.

The word *power* in its Greek form means "ability" and "capacity." When the word power is used in this section of the handbook, it refers to the knowledge individuals have, as well as to their capacity to choose wisely. In other words, a deliberate conscious decision is made to select one of three possible ways to act. The caregiver can give all the power over to the person for whom he or she is caring (YOU style). The caregiver can collaborate with others to make decisions and share the decision-making power (WE style). Or the caregiver can keep all the power and simply make the decisions (I style).

Because Alzheimer's disease will involuntarily change a person's behavior, the caregiver can easily feel helpless to make rational decisions and to understand the loved one's behavior in a rational way. Conflict and tension can be experienced among family members who have different ideas about what would be the best course of action. When a caregiver is in the midst of confusion, it is very difficult to be deliberate about decisions that have to be made.

For this reason, it is important that a caregiver have some objective way to view situations and arrive at decisions. I was delighted when Pat and Connie asked me to develop the three styles so that caregivers could think about the choices they have to make in some simple uncomplicated manner.

It was even more enlightening for us to discover that, although caregivers will act using all three styles, a pattern emerges when dealing with a person with Alzheimer's disease. Caregivers who were most successful in balancing their caregiving tasks seemed to use the YOU style most often when a person with Alzheimer's disease was in the early-to-mild stage of the disease. Caregivers used the WE style most often when a person with Alzheimer's disease was in the moderate stage of the disease, and they used the I style most often in the severe stage of the disease.

I am hopeful that the way the information is organized in this section will assist caregivers to feel comfortable about the decisions that will need to be made. The welfare and best interest of the person with Alzheimer's disease, as well as the caregiver's best interest, will require the caregiver to change the amount of power he holds on to or lets go of as the disease progresses. There is comfort in knowing you have explored all the options when you have reflected on the three styles.

Discover Your Preferred Style

To learn about your preferred style, you will need to tabulate the number of times you circled the numbers 1, 2, or 3 after each of the stories in Part III. A worksheet is provided for you on page 47. Once you have a total, you will learn how often you selected each of the three distinct styles.

The styles take into consideration the amount of control or power that is kept or given to others in any given situation. You have only three choices!

You can give the loved one with dementia all the power and act as a resource person to her. This is what you did each time you selected the #1 in the stories. Number one represents the YOU style.

You can collaborate with others—the person with Alzheimer's disease, family members, and health care personnel—to decide how to best meet some of your needs as a caregiver and the needs of the person with dementia. This is what you did each time you selected the #2 in the stories. Number two represents the WE style.

You can keep all the decision-making power. This is the choice you made each time you selected #3 in the stories. Number three represents the I style.

As you read through the descriptions of each style, you will recognize not only yourself, but the viewpoints of other family members or friends. Our hope is that the three styles will allow you to better understand the different perspectives on an issue and provide you with a way to communicate with others. Often, you will find that while you cannot change situations or events, you can change the way you think—and thus act—in them.

Understanding the styles can help:
1. Caregivers reflect on and learn about their "preferred style" of caregiving
2. Family members understand their different perspectives regarding how to best provide care
3. Families and health care providers keep the lines of communication open by asking objective questions about which style is the best to use for the loved one and for those providing care

Remember: There are always three choices!

The YOU Style (# 1)

The **caregiver allows** the loved one to lead . . . and acts as a resource person to the loved one.

In those stories where you selected a YOU response, you were acting as an advocate for the loved one with Alzheimer's disease. As long as the person was able to make the decisions for himself or herself and make good choices, you supported and encouraged the individual. You took your lead in acting from the loved one affected by the disease and served as a resource person to help him maintain an independent lifestyle as long as possible.

You can be encouraging and reassuring to others as the caregiver did in Story #5, when Karen was told she would have to retire. You probably reminded yourself often that, even though the person for whom you are caring may have lost her memory, the individual has not lost her mind. (See Story #5: How Should We Handle The News That It's Dementia?)

A person who works out of the YOU style focuses on the best each person has to offer life. You use skills of active listening, effective communication, and are sensitive to the feelings of others as well as your own feelings. You are not afraid to ask for what you need and tell others about your anxieties, apprehensions, feelings, and needs, as the caregiver did in Story #1, when she told her sister, "I am at my wits end." (See Story #1: Why Can't Mother Remember?)

You are able to allow others to express their feelings in an atmosphere of respect, and all topics are open for discussion. You can be patient and accept people where they are, like the children did in Story #3, when they resolved to wait for their father and mother to make some decisions about seeking professional counseling. (See Story #3: Is This the Person I Married?)

Your comfort in expressing feelings frees other persons to tell you their fears, their doubts, and their hopes for the present and the future. Sensitive topics can be discussed—sometimes with great emotional expression.

In unexpected situations, you tend to be spontaneous. You might use humor or creative solutions to diffuse or reflect tension. Recall how the two sisters in Story #4 told the mother, who forgot that she had given her daughter money, that they had won the lottery. Or recall how the caregiver in Story #10 had her mother's car towed and impounded when she forgot where she left it—rather than insist that she not drive. (See Story #4: Is It Okay If I Don't Tell the Truth? and Story #10: Where Are the Keys?)

Rather than tell the loved one what to do, you can be an observer. You might make mental notes and even record behavior patterns for the purpose of giving an accurate assessment of what is happening to the loved one for whom you are giving care.

You will refrain from doing things for persons that they can do for themselves and will encourage them to be independent as much as possible. You will help them maintain their dignity.

In this style of caregiving, you will be viewed by others as accessible, easy going, and comfortable with life's daily problems. Your skill in this style will serve you well when people are in the early-to-mild stage of dementia and can still communicate their wants and needs.

A pitfall of the YOU style is that you may empathize with the individual for whom you are caring and be unable to make objective decisions. As the disease takes over the person's mind and body, it can be difficult for you to view the changes and not take them to heart, as the daughter was tempted to do in Story #2, when her father was being unreasonable and refused to go to the assisted living facility. Having a clear-headed friend whom you can ask to help you when difficult decisions need to be made will be one way you can avoid this pitfall. Developing the skill of distinguishing fact from feeling is another way to avoid this pitfall. (See Story #2: How Can He Be So Insensitive?)

The YOU style:

- Acts as an advocate and resource person
- Encourages others
- Focuses on "positive qualities"
- Is an active listener
- Communicates effectively
- Is sensitive to the feelings of others
- Asks for what he or she needs
- Remains comfortable while discussing sensitive topics
- Can observe without interfering
- Is viewed as accessible by others
- Can become too emotionally involved
- Can find it difficult to make tough decisions

The WE style (#2)

The needs of both the caregiver and the loved one with dementia are equally considered. The caregiver keeps veto power to make ultimate decisions if the loved one is in danger.

In the stories where you selected a WE response, you most likely began to observe that, as much as you would like your loved one to have complete control over his or her life, more and more situations were calling for you to become actively involved. You were called to act as a negotiator in trying to get some of your needs met as well as meeting the needs of the person for whom you were giving care.

The Caregivers in Story #15 and in Story #14 realized that the best solution was to enlist the services of home health care so that the caregivers could find respite from being on call 24 hours a day. The mother and daughter, in Story #7, were willing to seek help from an Alzheimer's support group to gain perspective and balance in their lives. (See Story #15: Should a Caregiver Be On Call 24/7?, Story #14: Is There Caregiver Abuse?, and Story #7: Would My Mother Become Violent with Her Own Sister?)

The person working in the WE style will ask himself or herself the question: "What can my loved one still do, in spite of his or her diminished mental and physical capabilities?" The certified public accountant and his wife in Story #6 were willing to answer the question when they realized it was time to get a geriatric assessment. They wanted to know how they could continue to celebrate that which was not diminished, rather than focus on that which was being lost. (See Story #6: How Do I Know If Something Is Wrong?)

When you are in the WE style, you know clearly when you are unable to let the loved one have his or her desires. If the person is ever in physical or emotional danger, is being abusive or out-of-control, and you are unable to reason with him, you retain veto power to make direct, firm decisions that will keep the person safe. The caregiver in Story #12 realized one way to avoid being alone with her parents and subjected to their anger was to take them to places where they would be around more people. In public, their natural need for socialization would give them a chance to think about others and not focus on their own troubles. (See Story #12: Who Does the Changing?)

You are willing to share your time, talents, and treasures—all the while realizing that others can have opinions or ideas about caregiving that differ from yours. You believe once everyone has had a say, the most appropriate form of action can emerge when the options are viewed against the goal at hand. Henry and his wife in Story #13 were willing to make the generous offer to bring Henry's mom to their home when she could no longer take care of herself. The family in Story #16 was eager to be part of the care plan monitoring Ernie more closely when he needed activity. (See Story #13: How Was I To Know? and Story #16: Should We Use Restraints or Medication?)

You can be very attentive to the wishes and concerns of other family members and involve them as much as possible in understanding Alzheimer's disease and ways to care for the person as the disease progresses. You rely on experts in the field to assist you in your task of caregiving. The caregiver in Story #18 was relieved to learn about the Medicare Catastrophic Coverage Act that protected him from losing all his assets to pay for his wife's care. (See Story #18: Who Needs Help— The Caregiver or the Person with Dementia?)

A pitfall of the WE style can be that, in your concern that everyone has a say in matters, it may take too long to reach final decisions. This may become problematic if the person with Alzheimer's disease is becoming a source of danger to himself or others, is abusive, or is unreasonable. You might not act quickly enough if immediate and decisive decisions need to be made.

The WE style:
- Acts as a negotiator
- Understands the need for socialization
- Shares time, talents, treasures freely
- Expects different viewpoints and opinions
- Expects to take the lead sometimes and give the lead over at times

- Understands rights and responsibilities
- Relies on outside resources and experts
- Is comfortable delegating tasks
- May take a long time in coming to group decisions
- May want to keep all options open without coming to closure

The I style (#3)

The caregiver takes the lead and provides a plan of action. In those stories where you selected an *I* response, you were able to—and preferred to—use direct, authoritative approaches when working with other people. You like to have clear guidelines and limits to activities and feel comfortable taking the lead or control. You like things to be precise and accurate. This can work to your advantage or against you, as it did in Story #19, when Janice became frustrated trying to get her mother to recognize her. (See Story #19: Can You Accept Me For Who I Am Today?)

You frequently expect that others will respond positively to your lead and your good judgment and most of the time they do, seeing you as a very competent caregiver. In Story #8, after listening to the pros and cons of letting Pearl take the trial drug for her catastrophic reactions, Pearl's sons will most likely regain confidence that Charles has Pearl's best interests in mind. (See Story #8: Who Has Power of Attorney?)

You tend to be systematic in your approach and like to develop plans and outlines that will lead to a predictable outcome. You can be highly organized and find joy in ordering situations or people who appear to be in chaos. In Story #9, the caregiver found the most peace in moving her dad to a nursing home in Florida where she could continue to monitor his situation. Once she acted and moved her father, her brother also moved to Florida. (See Story #9: Whose Rights Prevail?)

Your skill in this style will serve you well when people are in crisis, when events are being planned for the first time, when structures need to be established, and when limits need to be set. You tend to be independent and objective and will be called upon to make the tough decisions when persons for whom you are caring can be a danger to themselves or others.

You might be the person who will say to the family of a loved one who is dying: "Look, we only have three choices. We can prolong life by inserting the feeding tube. We can make Dad comfortable and pain free and allow the dying process to proceed, or we can get another opin-

ion and buy some time before an ultimate decision needs to be made."
(See Story #20: To Hold On or To Let Go?)

A pitfall of the I style is that, in your concern for structure and
sometimes detail, others can see you as too busy, or too independent,
and they can feel as if you don't need them. They will hesitate to get
involved or believe you have everything under control and do not need
or want their help.

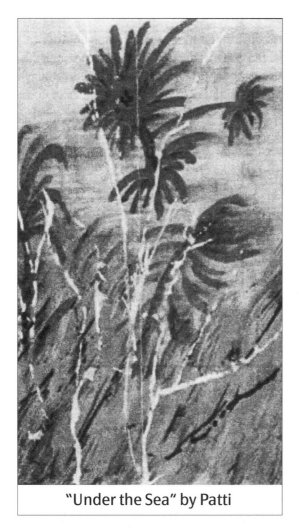

"Under the Sea" by Patti

Patti's zest for life and her love of arts and crafts have given her
the material to assist her in creating many beautiful pieces. All
Memories in the Making artists' works are created entirely by the
individual artist, with no assistance from anyone else. Most have
never painted before having Alzheimer's disease.

You can find that it is difficult for you to delegate responsibilities to others and trust that the job will be done as well as you can do it. This will give other persons the feeling that you are micro-managing and that their expertise is not appreciated. Telling others your thoughts, plans, and feelings and asking them for their opinions and help will keep the lines of communication open.

The I style:
- Uses direct, authoritative approaches
- Likes guidelines and limits
- Feels comfortable taking the lead
- Is highly organized and attentive to details
- Uses clear judgment and rationales
- Is systematic
- Can be counted on in times of crises
- Can be seen as too independent
- Has difficulty in delegating tasks

Learning Which Style Fits Best

If you are like most people, you probably have selected caregiving styles that fall under each of the three columns. It is valuable for caregivers to recognize that all three styles will come into play:

- Within any one day
- At certain times in the progression of the dementia
- In the way situations can be viewed and handled

One style—the column in which you have the most choices of YOU, WE, or I is your preferred style. It can become dominant when:

- You are involved in a conflict
- You feel overwhelmed
- You are involved in a new situation
- You are tired or haven't been taking care of yourself
- You have little time to think what would be best for you as the caregiver and the person for whom you are caring

It is during these times that it can be productive to reflect and understand the differences in the YOU, WE, and I styles. Are you going to take control and be comfortable with your decision? Will you need to "let go" and take your lead from the loved one; or will you need to enlist the help of others to accomplish what is needed? Sometimes your preferred style is not the most appropriate or effective way to respond to a situation. The healthy caregiver stops and thinks about what is best for himself or herself and for the person for whom he or she is caring *before responding or acting*.

Caregivers find it productive to use the YOU style when their loved one is in the early-to-mild stage of Alzheimer's disease or related dementia.

- The YOU style tends to work best during the early-to-mild stage of a person's dementia, when he or she can still make judgments and is aware of what is happening—even during times of forgetfulness.
- The YOU style allows the caregiver to give the loved one power to have control over his or her own life.
- The YOU style lets the caregiver yield to the needs of the loved one and give the person the dignity of his or her own choices.
- The YOU style is healthy for all concerned as long as the individual with Alzheimer's disease is safe and the caregiver understands the changes that are occurring.
- The YOU style is the only style a caregiver can have in the early stages of Alzheimer's if the loved one is strong willed and will not listen to others.

NOTE: As the capabilities of the person with dementia change—ever so slowly—the caregiver will need to take more responsibility in caregiving and shift to the WE and/or I styles as needed.

Caregivers find it productive to use the WE style when their loved one is in the moderate stage of Alzheimer's disease or related dementia.

- The WE style tends to work best during the moderate stage of a person's dementia and when the caregiver has been educated to know what to expect as the brain changes. The caregiver is in a better position to see that both he or she and the loved one get some of their needs met.
- In the WE style, the caregiver seeks resources for the person with dementia and for himself or herself.
- In the WE style, family members are involved as much as possible in understanding the disease and seeking solutions to future questions. Families can schedule regular times to meet to discuss

progress and assign different family members the task of research-ing other resources and programs for support or knowledge about the disease.

* In the WE style, the caregiver lets the person with dementia be as self-sufficient as possible, but still holds the power in the relation-ship to make decisions for the safety and well-being of the person with dementia.

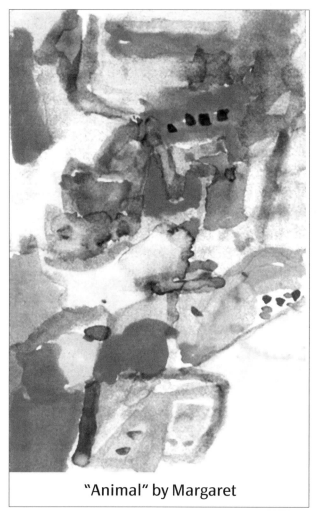

"Animal" by Margaret

Under the structured support of the Memories in the Making art program, Margaret has enjoyed painting, and she is especially inspired by works of Paul Klee. She explains that she had a Paul Klee painting in her home as a young girl. The picture is a message from a person who is striving to maintain her dignity and identity . . . despite the losses experienced.

Caregivers find it productive to use the I style when their loved one is in the severe stage of Alzheimer's disease or related dementia.

- The I style tends to work best during the later or severe stage of a person's dementia, when he or she is no longer able to make decisions.
- In the I style, the caregiver acts upon the desires of the loved one, which were discussed prior to this stage.
- In the I style, the caregiver has the power to make the end-of-life decisions for the person with Alzheimer's disease or related dementia.
- The I style works best if the loved one is in danger, is abusive, exhibits out-of-control behaviors, or is incapable of making rational decisions.
- The I style is used when time, resources, or personnel to give care have become depleted.

If you take the opportunity to stop and think before you act, you will have a better chance of being a very healthy caregiver.

Alzheimer's Disease: Changes in the Brain

Meet Roger A. Brumback, MD

My interest in dementia began with my work as the Chief of the Neurology Service at the Fargo, North Dakota VA Medical Center, where I had a number of patients with Parkinson's disease who also had signs of dementia. Subsequently, in 1983, I became involved in performing brain autopsies for the Alzheimer's Disease Research Center at the University of Rochester Medical Center.

These positions were but two of the stops in my diverse medical career. After graduating in 1971, in the inaugural class of the Pennsylvania State University College of Medicine at the Milton S. Hershey Medical Center, I trained in the pediatrics residency training program of the Johns Hopkins Hospital. Then, after training in neurology at Washington University in St. Louis and at the National Institutes of Health (NIH), I took the position in Fargo, where my research involved muscular dystrophy.

However, I became interested in dementia based upon my dealing with Parkinson's disease clinic patients. Then, when I decided to get residency training in anatomic pathology and neuropathology at the University of Rochester, I had the opportunity to work in one of the first NIH-supported dementia research programs.

After completing that pathology training, I was recruited to head the neuropathology programs at the University of Oklahoma Health Sciences Center and the Oklahoma City VA Medical Center. Working with the Oklahoma City Chapter of the Alzheimer's Association, I was able to get the Oklahoma legislature to provide an annual appropriation to support a brain bank and dementia autopsy program. This helped to jump-start several research laboratories and gave impetus to efforts to develop an Alzheimer's disease clinical center. After several years of discussion, the U.S. Congress provided a nearly $1 million annual appropriation for the Oklahoma City VAMC to develop such a clinical center with the purpose of providing medical care, education, and research that would allow improved caregiving for Alzheimer's disease patients.

It was then that my interest turned to developing programs to help the Alzheimer's disease patients and their families cope with the progression of this disorder. At the same time, I joined the board of directors of the Oklahoma City Alzheimer's Association and ascended to the position of president, where I was able to expedite the merger of the Oklahoma City and Tulsa chapters. In order to help educate the community about Alzheimer's disease, I was a frequent speaker at support groups and community organizations. I also undertook a weekly column (entitled "Ask Dr. B.") for the senior's page of the local Norman, Oklahoma newspaper.

In January 2001, I moved to Omaha to take the position of Chairman of the Department of Pathology at the Creighton University School of Medicine. In Omaha, I found a welcoming Alzheimer's Association chapter (and I now serve on the board of directors.) A part of that welcome included asking me to collaborate on this book project for caregivers.

In preparing this book, we decided that this section should be in the same question and answer format as my successful newspaper column. We hope this section will help everyone understand what changes happen in the brain when someone has Alzheimer's disease or related dementia, thus making us better caregivers, family members, and friends. We will understand that the dignity of the person remains and should be nurtured and stimulated so that some good times, quiet times, and happy times can still be enjoyed. Even though the brain is damaged as the disease progresses, the dignity of the person remains.

The person should not be "set aside" as if he or she does not know what is going on . . . or is not capable of functioning as a person.

So, imagine yourself sitting in my office, asking me the following questions in your search to better understand what is going on with Alzheimer's disease and related dementia. Sit back and relax, have a cup of tea—green tea if you have it—and listen to the answers.

A DIALOGUE WITH DR. ROGER A. BRUMBACK

Q: Doesn't everyone get senile as they get older?

A: There is a great myth in America and Western Europe that all older people normally lose their thinking and reasoning abilities and become "senile." The cut off time seems to be 65 years of age—after that age, the brain just can't work right any more. Thus, everyone over age 65 years is considered to be senile. Of course, the mandatory retirements around that age only emphasize the fact that older people can't be productive anymore. This idea actually began in the mid-nineteenth century in Germany as socialistic programs were being introduced. Politicians decided that those over age 65 years were senile and no longer mentally competent to work. Medical researchers then undertook investigations to determine what happened to the brain to cause this senility. Some investigators, who looked under the microscope at samples from autopsied brains of people over the age of 65 years, found what they called "senile plaques" and thought that these caused the mental deterioration.

In the early 1900s, one of these researchers, Alois Alzheimer, studied a woman with memory loss beginning at age 51 years that progressed over 4 1/2 years to apathy, loss of speech, incontinence, and death. At autopsy, Alzheimer found in the brain the same senile plaques and neurofibrillary tangles that other investigators had found in people over age 65 years. Thus, Alzheimer said that this lady suffered from premature senility (she had become senile before the expected age of 65 years when everyone normally became senile) and called the disease *presenile dementia*. Later, his boss Emil Kraeplin named this rare condition causing people to become senile before the expected age of 65 years, *Alzheimer's disease*.

Of course, we now understand that Alzheimer's disease can affect people at any age from 30 years to 100 years, and we also know that the myth of senility is untrue. Any thoughtful consideration of the many accomplishments of friends, relatives, acquaintances, or public figures who are over age 65 years debunks the myth of senility.

Research studies have also shown that people do not lose thinking and reasoning ability as they age. What does change over time is the speed of all activity. With age we all slow down. For example, in the Olympics, there were no sprinters or swimmers over the age of 50 years. In fact, a number of years ago, it was considered remarkable that at age 35 years, the American sprinter Carl Lewis could still compete in the Olympics, although not in any of the sprints. Thus, when 20-year-olds and 60-year-olds are compared on IQ tests, the 20-year-olds will always score better on the tests that have a time limit for completion; 20-year-olds get done quickly, while 60-year-olds often have not completed the task at the end of the allowed time. On the other hand, in tests of information, knowledge, reasoning, and logic, which are not timed, the 60-year-olds score better than the 20-year-olds. Thus, as we all age, we slow down, but our ability to reason improves. This only makes sense: How many 20-year-olds are able to make the wisest decisions?

Unfortunately, since we live in a "sound bite" society in which quick decisions and answers are more important than good decisions, the slow (but carefully reasoned) decisions of elderly people are often considered evidence of "senility."

Q: What is dementia?

A: Dementia is a medical problem characterized by the progressive loss of intellectual and cognitive abilities sufficient to result in impaired social and work functioning. Although the term dementia is usually applied to elderly people, dementia can also occur in younger adults. Dementia is not really a disease, but is a symptom of something going wrong in the brain. In other words, dementia is what you witness in the patient's behavior, but what is happening in the brain is the disease causing the dementia.

Sometimes the disease causing dementia is actually a treatable condition. In fact, out of 100 people consulting a family physician about the symptoms of dementia, almost half of them may have a treatable condition (and treatment could stop or even reverse the dementia). There are many potentially treatable diseases and conditions that can cause dementia, and a complete medical and neurologic examination is necessary to identify the possible causes. For example, low thyroid hormone (called hypothyroidism) can produce a dementia that can be completely cured by taking thyroid hormone tablets. This thorough evaluation for treatable

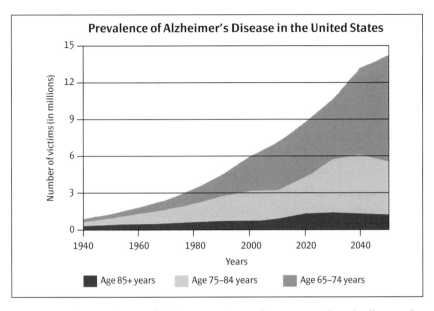

FIGURE 1. The prevalence of Alzheimer's disease has increased markedly over the past 50 years, and will continue to do so for the next 50.

causes of dementia requires extensive testing and can be rather expensive. On the other hand, some causes of dementia are irreversible and ultimately fatal because the nerve cells in the brain die. These causes of dementia are called *neurodegenerative disorders* and Alzheimer's disease is one of many different neurodegenerative disorders that include Pick's disease, Lewy body disease, and many others.

Alzheimer's disease is becoming more prevalent as our life expectancy increases. For example, one out of every two people over the age of 85 years will have Alzheimer's disease. Currently, there are over 6 million victims of this disorder in the United States and, by the year 2030, estimates suggest that number of victims will double to about 12 million (**Figure 1**).

Q: Is it true that some things are only done by certain parts of the brain?

A: Although the brain weighs only about 3 pounds and could fit comfortably in the palm of the hand, it is the most important part of the body. The brain is different from other organs of the body in that every nerve cell in the brain does something unique that only that nerve cell can do and no other nerve cell can do. This is in contrast, for example, to the liver, since the left half of the liver does the same as the right half of the liver and every liver cell does the same as every other liver cell. The same is true for the kidneys, in that the left kidney does the same as the right kidney, and a person can even lose one kidney because the remaining kidney can take over and do everything. However, in the brain, every part has a specific function, and all the parts must work together for the brain to work correctly. Loss of any part of the brain results in loss of that function, because no other part of the brain can take over or perform that function.

The brain consists of three major parts (**Figure 2**). The large wrinkled part that sits on top is called the *cerebrum*, which is the thinking part of the brain. Beneath the cerebrum in back is the *cerebellum*, which functions to keep the body balanced upright (for example, in walking or climbing). In front of the cerebellum is a thick cable system called the *brainstem*, which connects everything together, including connecting the cerebrum to the cerebellum, to the spinal cord, and to the eyes,

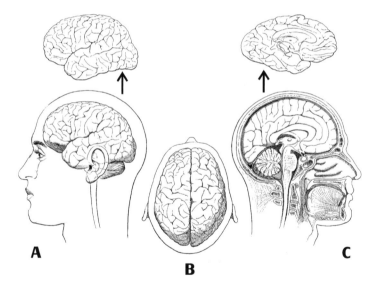

FIGURE 2. Drawings of the brain in relationship to the head. (A) The left side of the head with the brain inside (below) and the left cerebral hemisphere separately (above). The outside surface of the cerebral hemisphere is wrinkled with mounds of brain tissue (called *gyri*) separated by spaces (called *sulci*). The general appearance of the brain surface is the same for everyone, but the detailed arrangement of the wrinkles is unique for each individual, just like fingerprints. (B) The head and brain from above shows that the brain is divided in the center (middle) into left and right cerebral hemispheres. (C) The head and brain cut through the center (midline) showing the middle of the head and brain (below) and the cerebral hemisphere separately (above).

ears, nose, throat, and all the nerves in the body. (For more information see Appendix I.)

Q: What happens in the brain of the person diagnosed with Alzheimer's disease?

A: Alzheimer's disease causes the progressive death of nerve cells in the cerebral hemispheres of the brain. The nerve cells do not all die at once, but instead a slow death march moves from one area of the brain to the next area.

The first area in which nerve cells die is the *hippocampus* of the limbic lobe (**Figure 3**), which is in the center of the cerebral hemisphere; the hippocampus is the memory area of the brain. All memory is cataloged and recorded by the hippocampus (**Figure 4**).

Because the hippocampus controls memory, the first symptom relates to memory loss. However, the rest of the brain functions normally, so the person still moves and feels things, still sees, still hears, and still integrates information. Because judgment, reasoning, and social skills are still functioning normally, the person can develop compensatory coping strategies to deal with the memory problems (for example, making lists or relying on others to remember).

Thus, in this beginning stage of the disease process, no one will be aware of the problem because of these compensations, and the person will appear normal and never consult a physician. Nonetheless, researchers have shown that very extensive neuropsychological testing can demonstrate this memory loss, which has been called *benign senile forgetfulness*.

Limbic Lobe

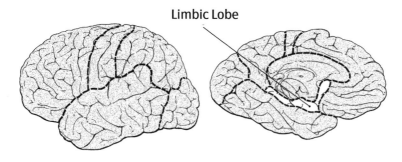

FIGURE 3. The left cerebral hemisphere of the brain viewed from the outside and from the center showing the limbic lobe that contains the hippocampus which is the memory area of the brain.

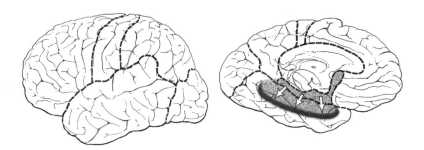

FIGURE 4. The shaded area indicates the site of the initial damage in Alzheimer's disease involving the limbic lobe hippocampus resulting in memory loss.

I first noticed I was forgetting things more often especially when I would put something away and then the next day have to look for it. I would go grocery shopping and go down aisle one and then aisle two. When I was at the end of aisle two, I found myself going back down aisle one again. This would happen quite often. Sometimes I would go shopping and I would forget the coupons and have to drive back home to get them. Many times my daughters would phone, and I would mistakenly call them by their wrong name. To cover up my mistake I would say, "Oh, you sound just like your sister!"

At my last check-up the doctor asked if I had any new problems since my last visit. That's when I told him about my memory problem. The doctor gave me a simple quiz and asked me who our president was and if I knew where I was right now. He asked me to spell words and recall items he just mentioned. I got all those questions right.

The doctor said most people past 60 years old could have memory loss and recommended an MRI test. He then prescribed a pill called Aricept®, which was to be taken once a day. Boy are they expensive! I have noticed a big improvement since taking this pill.

—Anna, patient with dementia,
age 87 (See Modified Cognitive Functioning Quiz
entitled "How Healthy Is Your Brain?" in Appendix 2.)

Q: As the disease progresses from the early-to-mild stage to the moderate stage what happens in the brain?

A: The Alzheimer's disease process is unrelenting and continues to destroy nerve cells, with the destruction spreading out over the brain like a wave ("a tidal wave of destruction"). From the hippocampus, this

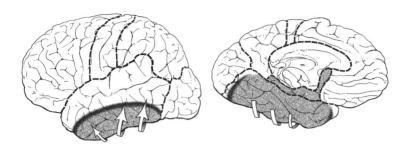

FIGURE 5. The wave of destruction from Alzheimer's disease spreads from the limbic lobe to involve the temporal lobe, resulting in problems with understanding words and using the correct words.

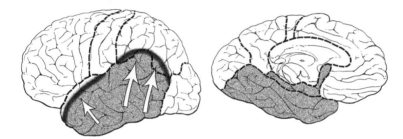

FIGURE 6. Once the wave of destruction from Alzheimer's disease has destroyed the temporal lobe, the person has problems communicating and becomes less interactive and more withdrawn.

destructive wave then spreads over the temporal lobe, causing the person to have trouble understanding words or expressing the correct words (Figures 5 and 6).

The problem with using or understanding words causes conflicts with others but also causes the individual to withdraw and communicate less. Also, because the frontal lobes are still intact, the person tries to judge why others do not seem to understand. An example could help to illustrate this problem:

An elderly husband and wife are sitting at the breakfast table as they do every morning, and the man is about to drink his coffee. He asks his wife to "pass the salt." She obliges, and he becomes angry. What he actually wanted was the sugar to put in his coffee, but because of the Alzheimer's disease damage to his temporal lobe, the word came out as "salt." He is angry because his wife has recently been responding to his requests like this everyday. Because his frontal lobe judgment and reasoning are still intact, he has been trying to figure out why she is doing this and seems to have the answer: she knows he has high blood pressure and if he takes in more salt he will die and she can collect the life insurance.

The brain changes of Alzheimer's disease affects his ability to interact with his wife and is making him more suspicious of everything his wife does. At the same time, the wife is becoming increasingly unhappy that her husband is so irritable when she does exactly what he asks her to do. The solution is for the wife to recognize that her husband is having problems using the correct words, to anticipate his requests, and to respond appropriately (i.e., passing the sugar to him even though he says "salt"). Unfortunately, patients with Alzheimer's disease rarely come for medical attention at this stage and families do not obtain information about this caregiving solution.

Q: What happens as the disease progresses through the moderate stage of Alzheimer's?

A: The wave of destruction then spreads out over the parietal lobes (**Figure 7**). When this occurs, the person loses the ability to integrate visual, sound (auditory), and body sensation information. This is the stage at which the individual has trouble dressing, gets lost or is disoriented, and cannot figure out how to use objects. For example, in this stage, the individual will sit at a dinner table but not be able to start eating because the visual information about food and utensils cannot be integrated. The person needs help to use the knife, fork, and spoon properly.

The biggest problem seems to be in integrating the visual information so that, although the person appears unable to eat, placing the utensils in the person's hand (providing the body sensation of the utensil in the hand) will be enough for him or her to begin eating. The person also has great difficulty asking for things (or for help) because the destructive process of Alzheimer's disease has already passed through and devastated the temporal lobe speech areas.

This is also the stage of the disease process in which driving becomes problematic because the individual gets lost and cannot integrate all the visual and audible information of the environment with the proper body sensation of the steering wheel and floor pedals. Patients generally consult physicians for evaluation when the parietal lobes become involved by the Alzheimer's disease destructive process. No longer are the frontal lobe compensatory mechanisms sufficient, and family mem-

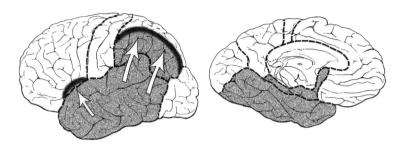

FIGURE 7. When the wave of destruction enters the parietal lobe, the patient experiences disorientation and difficulties with complex tasks. By this stage of moderate severity, most patients will have consulted a physician and received the diagnosis.

bers and acquaintances become aware that a problem requiring medical evaluation exists.

Q: What happens as the disease progresses into the severe stage of Alzheimer's?

A: Once the parietal lobes have been devastated, the Alzheimer's disease process then moves into the frontal lobes **(Figure 8)**. Once the frontal lobes are damaged, the person loses the ability to interact properly. This is the stage at which many patients can no longer be managed by caregivers at home. The individuals lose judgment, reasoning, and social skills, and at this stage respond inappropriately and unacceptably, having lost much of their "civilized" behavior. For example:

> In the parietal lobe stage of Alzheimer's disease, the person could go out to a restaurant with the family, sit quietly, eat the meal (after some help from family members with the utensils and the food), and behave appropriately for such a social situation (although not remembering having eaten after the meal was over).
>
> However, in the frontal lobe stage of the disease, such a restaurant visit would be problematic because of the loss of judgment and any normal social inhibitions. A male with Alzheimer's disease might grab the breasts of a young waitress, a woman might feel warm and just strip off all her clothes to feel cool.

At varying times in the frontal lobe stage, the person can be very violent with rages or very docile, apathetic, and immobile. Touching

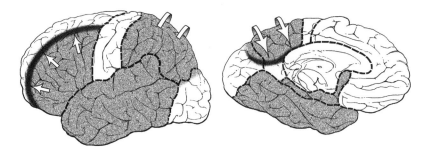

FIGURE 8. In the severe stage of Alzheimer's disease, the frontal lobe is devastated, and the patient loses judgment and normal social interaction.

(such as helping the person undress) can trigger violence to repel the contact, possibly injuring either the caregiver or the person with Alzheimer's disease.

In the end stages (**Figure 9**), the destructive process of Alzheimer's disease has killed nearly all the nerve cells of the cerebral hemispheres except the strip of motor cortex and the visual cortex, which is why in nursing homes, the main activity seems to be walking and pacing. In the final stages, even these brain areas are destroyed, and the individual will be bedridden and relatively unresponsive.

Q: What actually causes Alzheimer's disease?

A: Alzheimer's disease is the result of something killing nerve cells in the cerebral hemispheres of the brain. When the nerve cells die, they

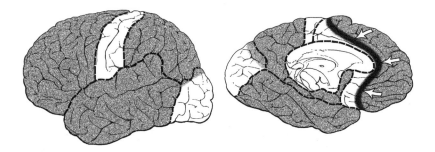

FIGURE 9. By the end stage of the disease, the wave of destruction has destroyed nearly all the cerebral hemisphere.

leave behind tombstones marking the site of their death. These tombstones are distinctive and are called *neurofibrillary tangles* and *senile neuritic amyloid plaques*. The tangles and plaques are readily seen under the microscope in samples from autopsy brains of victims of Alzheimer's disease.

So far, investigators have not discovered what causes the nerve cells to die in Alzheimer's disease. One early theory was that exposure to too much aluminum from cooking pots and soda cans caused the nerve cells to die. Although it is true that the plaques contain large amounts of aluminum, the aluminum does not cause them. Instead, because aluminum that gets into the body has to be carried by the blood stream to the kidneys for elimination in the urine, any blood containing aluminum that passes through the brain has the aluminum sucked out into preformed plaques.

It now appears that Alzheimer's disease is the result of many factors including a genetic susceptibility and many environmental and nutritional factors. Alzheimer's disease does seem to run in families, and this susceptibility allows the disease to occur in younger people in some families. Genetic factors are only one aspect of the susceptibility, however, because researchers have studied identical twins, who have the same genes but have different lifestyles and have gotten the disease at different ages (up to a decade apart). Dietary factors also seem to be important, as do hormonal levels. In addition, there appears to be an aspect of "use it or lose it" in the development of Alzheimer's disease. That is, people with Alzheimer's disease who are intellectually active seem to be able to stave off the development of the disease until much later in life than might otherwise have occurred.

Q: Is it true that the disease can actually go undetected for many years?

A: This question really raises two issues. As described above, Alzheimer's disease actually begins first in the hippocampus and affects memory. However, because the rest of the brain, particularly the frontal lobe, is not affected, the individual can compensate, and observers will not notice a problem. Thus, for a number of years, the disease process causes a problem, but the difficulty is hidden unless careful neuropsychological testing is performed. Only in a later stage, when speech problems or more likely when disorientation occurs, will the individual seek medical attention and be diagnosed with Alzheimer's disease. Thus, the disease seems to have been "hidden" for many years.

Another issue should be clarified, however—the preclinical stage of the disease process. To understand this aspect of Alzheimer's disease, it is necessary to describe something about the normal development of the brain. As the brain develops in utero inside the mother during gestation, nerve cells are formed. All nerve cells are produced by the 20th week of gestation, which is at the 4 1/2-month point or halfway to term (birth). At 20 weeks gestation, the brain weighs almost 2 ounces. From that point on, the nerve cells migrate to their final positions and start to make connections. By birth, the brain has increased in size to 1 pound because of the growth of the connecting branches of the nerve cells.

No new nerve cells can be formed, however, and the nerve cells must survive the process of birth (the head being banged through the small birth canal) and then all the illnesses and high fevers of childhood and the head trauma (the child hitting its head as it falls learning to walk, etc.). Because the loss of nerve cells could be catastrophic since each area of the brain has unique functions that cannot be performed by other areas, nature devised an "80% safety margin" in the brain (**Figure 10**). That is, for every nerve cell, four spare nerve cells exist, which means that generally humans only use 20% of their brain capacity. Using these extra nerve cells would not somehow make us smarter, because we need the extras as spares for all the nerve cells that are lost over our lifetime.

This is similar to the situation of the automobile that has a spare tire in the trunk. That spare can be lifesaving if the driver experiences a flat tire out in a deserted mountain pass in the middle of a massive winter snowstorm. But because the car only has one spare tire, the situation could still be perilous if the driver experienced another flat tire before reaching safety. In the brain, there are four spare nerve cells, because brain function must survive a lifetime of possible insults.

Researchers have found that over an 80-year lifetime, humans normally lose as many as 40% of the nerve cells (in other words, two out of a set of five nerve cells are lost, but three out of five remain). Fortunately, this means that two spares still remain to back up the main functioning nerve cell. In Alzheimer's disease, when the nerve cell destruction starts, there are still plenty of spare nerve cells. Thus, as a nerve cell dies, a spare will immediately take over as though nothing had happened. As nerve cells continue to die, however, there will be fewer and fewer spares to take over. Finally, when no spares are left and the main functioning nerve cell dies, the person will start to have problems. This is referred to as crossing the threshold of the 80% safety margin and is the beginning of the clinical stage of the disease process. Before that time, the disease is in the preclinical stage, which in the case of Alzheimer's disease (**Figure 10**) occurs over 20 to 30 years. Thus,

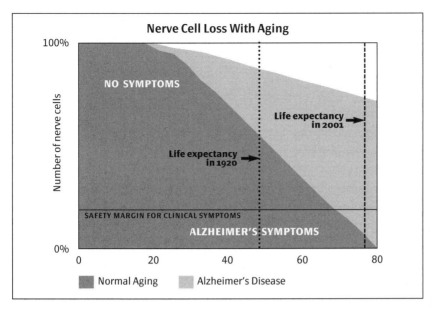

Nerve Cell Loss With Aging

Number of nerve cells

NO SYMPTOMS

Life expectancy in 2001

Life expectancy in 1920

SAFETY MARGIN FOR CLINICAL SYMPTOMS

ALZHEIMER'S SYMPTOMS

Normal Aging   Alzheimer's Disease

FIGURE 10. Normal aging is associated with loss of some neurons, but this loss never exceeds the threshold of the 80% safety margin for clinical symptoms. The nerve cell loss in Alzheimer's disease is accelerated with age and causes symptoms when enough nerve cells are lost. With the short life-expectancy before the advent of modern medical advances, most individuals died before the age of 50, but with life expectancy now nearing 80 years, people will live long enough to develop the symptoms of Alzheimer's disease.

Alzheimer's disease seems to have a long preclinical stage of about 20 to 30 years and a long early clinical stage (the benign senile forgetfulness) of about 10 years, before the individual comes to medical attention. Following diagnosis, Alzheimer's disease often progresses to death in about 7 to 10 years.

Q: Is Alzheimer's disease more common than it used to be?

A: Alzheimer's disease is a disorder in which the nerve cells of the brain die over many years. Thus, an individual has to live long enough for the disease to affect the brain. Before the middle of the twentieth century, the average life expectancy was less than 50 years. Now, average life expectancy exceeds 70 years, so that more people will live long enough to show the clinical stages of Alzheimer's disease. In addition, because women live longer than men, there will be slightly more women than men with Alzheimer's disease. Statisticians believe that, unless we find a cure for the disorder, there will be nearly 20 million victims in the United States when the baby-boomer generation reaches old age.

Q: How long does it take people to die of Alzheimer's disease?

A: Many people have described Alzheimer's disease as a "slow, living death" because of the progressive deterioration and loss of human abilities to interact normally. The early-to-mild stage of the disease can last for a variable number of years, and often, because of the ability of the brain to compensate, the individual goes undiagnosed during this period. Those individuals diagnosed in this stage of the disease do not progress into the next stage of the disease for 3 to 5 years, however. Nearly all patients are diagnosed by the moderate stage of the disease, and progression through this stage lasts for about 3 to 5 years. Because the median survival (the time by which half the patients die) is 7 years after diagnosis, many individuals will die before they reach the severe stage of the disease. Survival during the severe stage depends a lot on the quality of nursing care, because patients lose many of the self-care functions that prevent other illnesses. Alzheimer's disease is the underlying cause of death; that is, it weakens brain control of body systems and allows other illnesses to end the patient's life.

Q: Is there any treatment for Alzheimer's disease?

A: The issue of treatment is an important one and must be addressed in two ways—medical treatment and supportive therapy.

Q: What is the medical treatment for Alzheimer's disease?

A: Although the earliest symptom of Alzheimer's disease is memory loss, few individuals seek medical attention at this stage. Even if the Alzheimer's disease-associated memory loss could be identified at its onset, the side-effects of the medications which supercharge the few remaining nerve cells in the hippocampus could reduce the effectiveness of treatment. Actually, the compensatory mechanisms of the intact frontal lobe executive functions are often just as useful in social and occupational settings with fewer potential side effects.

By the time the disease has spread over the temporal lobe, language problems are added to the memory difficulties, and the temporal lobe language problems cannot be affected by the medications that super-charge the hippocampus. In addition, once language problems are prominent, fewer viable neurons remain in the hippocampus to be supercharged. By the time parietal lobe symptoms appear (the stage at which most patients present for medical evaluation), there are virtually no neurons in the hippocampus to respond to the supercharging medication. Thus, medication used to treat Alzheimer's disease memory loss used beyond the period of the discrete memory loss are either ineffective or produce mainly a placebo effect.

Q: What is supportive treatment for Alzheimer's disease?

A: Education of the affected individual, caregivers, family, and friends regarding both the lost and the preserved brain functions is part of a supportive therapy program. Instead of focusing on deficits, the focus should be on the preserved abilities and the development of compensatory strategies.

The search for preserved abilities can seem onerous, but it can be very rewarding. For example, nursing home patients with Alzheimer's disease and little remaining self-care abilities have been described as being able to play winning dominos, contract bridge, or checkers when placed at an already set-up game table. Another report described a former professional jazz musician, who near the end-stage of Alzheimer's disease, could still play remarkable jazz performances when his assembled trombone was positioned in his hand and the mouthpiece put up to his lips. Thus, it is important to identify those skills that remain and focus not on the loss of functions but the preserved functions and the person who remains.

Of course, the ideal solution would be to find a way to stop the nerve cell death while the disease is still in the preclinical stage. Many pharmaceutical companies are working hard to find such a treatment.

THE PROGRESSION OF ALZHEIMER'S DISEASE IN THE BRAIN FROM ROGER A. BRUMBACK, MD

What happens in the brain during the early-to-mild stage (generally a 3 to 5 year period)?

* The first area in which nerve cells die as a result of Alzheimer's disease is the memory area of the brain.

* Because judgment, reasoning, and social skills are still functioning normally, the person can develop compensatory coping strategies to deal with the memory problems.
* Thus, in the beginning stage of the disease process, no one will be aware of the problem because of these compensations and the person will appear normal and never consult a physician.

What happens as the disease progresses toward the moderate stage (generally a 3 to 5 year period)?

* The wave of destruction then spreads. This is the stage that the individual has trouble dressing, gets lost or disoriented, and cannot figure out how to use objects.
* This is also the stage of the disease process where driving becomes problematic because the individual cannot integrate all the visual and sound information of the environment with the proper body sensations of the steering wheel and floor pedals.
* This is the time that a patient generally consults a physician for an evaluation. Family members and acquaintances become aware that a problem requiring medical evaluation exists.

What happens as the disease progresses into the severe stage

* The person loses the ability to interact properly. This is the stage at which a patient can no longer be managed by caregivers at home. The person loses judgment, reasoning, and social skills.
* Since the median survival (the time by which half the patients die) is 7 years after diagnosis, an individual may die before reaching the Severe Stage of the disease.
* Survival during the Severe Stage depends a lot on the quality of nursing care since patients lose many of the self-care functions that prevent other illnesses. Alzheimer's disease is the underlying cause of death; that is, it weakens the brain control of body systems and allows other illnesses to end the patient's life.

A DOCTOR'S PERSPECTIVE: PRESERVED SKILLS

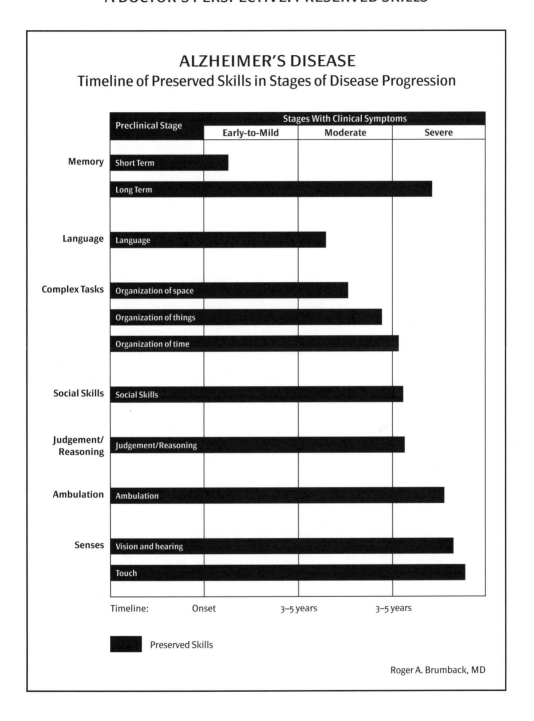

ALZHEIMER'S DISEASE
Timeline of Preserved Skills in Stages of Disease Progression

	Preclinical Stage	Stages With Clinical Symptoms		
		Early-to-Mild	Moderate	Severe
Memory	Short Term			
	Long Term			
Language	Language			
Complex Tasks	Organization of space			
	Organization of things			
	Organization of time			
Social Skills	Social Skills			
Judgement/ Reasoning	Judgement/Reasoning			
Ambulation	Ambulation			
Senses	Vision and hearing			
	Touch			

Timeline: Onset   3–5 years   3–5 years

■ Preserved Skills

Roger A. Brumback, MD

Appendices

APPENDIX 1
Additional Information about the Brain

The cerebrum is the part that is important in understanding the problems in Alzheimer's disease. The cerebrum is the part of the brain in which all of our thoughts reside; it has an almost spherical shape and is divided in the center, so each half is termed a *cerebral hemisphere*.

Thus, there are two cerebral hemispheres: a right cerebral hemisphere and a left cerebral hemisphere. The surface layers of the cerebral hemispheres contain all the nerve cells and are called the *cerebral cortex*. The cerebral hemispheres can be further subdivided into different *lobes,* which perform different specific functions.

One of these lobes is the strip of the brain called the *paracentral* (or *sensorimotor*) lobe (or lobule). This part of the brain initiates all body movement and feels all body sensation. The sensorimotor lobe is divided in half, with the front half being the *motor cortex* and the back half (**Figure 11**) being the *sensory cortex*. The motor cortex generates all body movement, but does so in a cross-over manner: that is, the motor cortex of the left cerebral hemisphere moves the right side of the body,

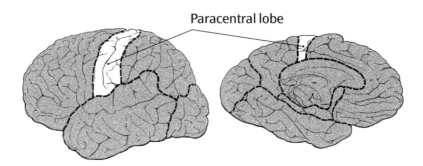

FIGURE 11. Paracentral (or sensorimotor) lobe of the brain, which controls body movement and feels body sensation.

and the right cerebral motor cortex moves the left side of the body. Just behind the motor cortex is the *sensory cortex*, where all body sensations are felt. Again, the left sensory cortex feels the right side of the body, and the right sensory cortex feels the left side of the body. The sensory cortex and motor cortex are adjacent to each other for an important reason: integration must exist between body movements and the sensations related to those movements. For example, when the sensory cortex feels the burning pain of touching a hot pan, it immediately instructs the adjacent motor cortex to send signals to move the hand away from the pan.

The back part of the cerebral hemispheres, called the *occipital lobe* (**Figure 12**), is dedicated to vision processing. Our eyes are like cameras, but the development of the film into pictures (images) occurs in the *visual cortex* of the occipital lobes. The visual cortex develops the pictures in real time so that we can see action as it occurs.

On the lower side of each cerebral hemisphere is a brain portion called the *temporal lobe* (**Figure 13**). The temporal lobes (also called the

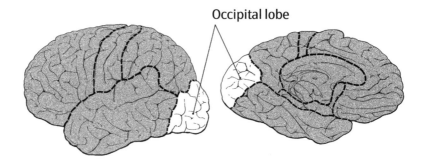

FIGURE 12. The occipital lobe of the brain controls vision.

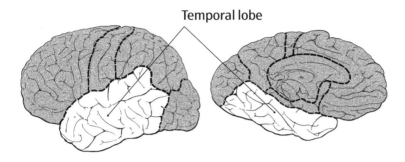
Temporal lobe

FIGURE 13. The temporal lobes of the brain process sound.

auditory cortex) are where the brain processes sound. The ears are receivers for sounds, which are then sent to the brain for interpretation. For humans, sounds consist of two important qualities: speech sounds (language) and nonspeech sounds (**Table 1**).

The left temporal lobe is specialized to interpret speech sounds and the right temporal lobe is specialized to process nonspeech sounds. To interpret speech sounds, the left temporal lobe has a "dictionary," containing all the information about the meanings of words, correct pronunciation, grammar, and usage. How many words are in this "dictionary" depends on environment and education. The right temporal lobe interprets all nonspeech sounds, such as music and environmental noises. The right temporal lobe also contributes to the understanding of speech by interpreting the tone, quality, volume, and melody of speech sounds (which are the emotional parts of speech sounds called *prosody*). Prosody is an important part of human communication, adding meaning and interest to the speech—anyone who has listened to a lecturer speak in monotone understands the importance of prosody. (Of note, in 1951, the comedian Stan Freberg produced a hit

TABLE 1. Comparison of the sound functions of the left and right temporal lobes

Left Temporal Lobe	Right Temporal Lobe
Interprets speech Contains dictionary of word meanings, correct pronunciation, rules of grammar	Interprets nonspeech sounds Interprets music and environmental noises Interprets tone, quality, volume, melody (prosody)

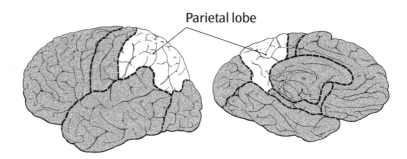

Parietal lobe

FIGURE 14. Parietal lobe is situated between the occipital, temporal, and para-central lobes and integrates vision, hearing, and body sensation.

record in which the only words were the names "John" and "Marsha" spoken with different inflections and tones.)

The *parietal lobe* (**Figure 14**) is the large area on the side of the brain that is situated between the visual cortex of the occipital lobe, the auditory cortex of the temporal lobe, and the sensory cortex of the sensorimotor lobe. This position allows the parietal lobe to integrate together information from vision, hearing, and body sensation about all those things we interact with in our environment. For example, when reaching into a pocket to get change, the coins will have a certain feel and sound as they clink together. The parietal lobe integrates this sensation information from the sensory cortex and the sound information from the temporal lobe to provide instructions to the hand to pick out the coins from other objects (such as keys) in the pocket. Then, when the handful of coins is brought out of the pocket and displayed, the parietal lobe integrates the visual information to confirm that the desired coins were correctly removed from the pocket.

The largest part of the cerebral hemisphere is in front and is called the *frontal lobe* (**Figure 15**). The frontal lobe is the most "human" part of the brain, and it differentiates humans from lower primates (chimpanzees and monkeys) and other animals. In fact, chimpanzees have all the same parts of the brain as humans, even areas that look similar to the speech and nonspeech areas of the temporal lobe. The reason a human forehead goes straight upwards and a chimpanzee's slants backward, however, is the human frontal lobe: *the frontal lobes make us human.* The frontal lobe contains all the rules of behavior that allow us to interact and live together in a society. The frontal lobe controls our ability to know right from wrong and socially acceptable or unac-

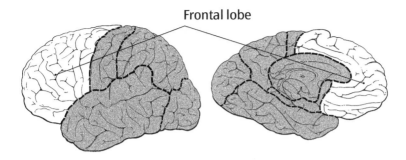

Frontal lobe

FIGURE 15. The frontal lobe is the largest part of the cerebral hemisphere and is responsible for judgment, reasoning, logic, insight/foresight, self-awareness, social rules and behavior, and control of the rest of the brain (executive control function).

ceptable behavior. The frontal lobe is responsible for reasoning, judgment, logic, insight/foresight, self-awareness, and the control of the rest of the brain (something called *executive control function*). During several decades in the middle of the twentieth century, a barbaric procedure called *frontal lobotomy* (in which the frontal lobe on each side was cut out) was used to treat schizophrenia and other mental illnesses. Removing the frontal lobes caused the patients to become "zombie-like" and lose all their human social qualities. The importance of human frontal lobes can be illustrated by considering how differently a human and a chimpanzee would react to finding a stamped, sealed, addressed envelope on the ground in front of a U.S. mailbox. The human would pick up the envelope and place it in the mailbox, whereas a chimpanzee would play with the envelope and probably crumple it, tear it, and mouth it but not place it in the mailbox.

APPENDIX 2
Self-Assessment: How Healthy Is Your Brain?

Invite someone to help you with this task.

Basic Instruction	Item for Scoring	Major Cognitive Function Tested
1. Ask a series of questions about time and place. Give yourself one point for each correct answer.	1. What year is it? 2. What season are we in? 3. What month are we in? 4. What is today's date? 5. What day of the week is it? 6. What state are we in? 7. What country are we in? 8. What city (town) are we in? 9. What is the approximate time? 10. What is your home address?	Memory
2. Name three common objects (examples include "cup," "orange," "chair," "dollar bill," "cap"); pronounce each word carefully; have the person immediately repeat all three and record success. Repeat each until person learns all three and is told to remember these words for the future.	11. First object? 12. Second object? 13. Third object?	Learning, Immediate Recall, Understanding Words
3. Alternate tasks: Serial 6's (starting at 100 serially subtract 6); stop after five answers. Or, spell the word "brain" backwards.	14. 94 15. 88 16. 82 17. 76 18. 70 14. N 15. I 16. A 17. R 18. B	Concentration, Arithmetic

Basic Instruction	Item for Scoring	Major Cognitive Function Tested
4. Recall the three object words memorized earlier.	19. First object? 20. Second object? 21. Third object?	Delayed Memory
5. Show two objects (examples include "pen," "watch," "pencil," "clock," "cup") and ask the person to name each.	22. First object 23. Second object	Naming
6. Ask the person to repeat a specific nonsense phrase.	24. "No ifs, ands, or buts."	Ability with words Following Instructions
7. Ask the person to follow a three-stage command. Place a piece of paper on a table and instruct the person to follow directions.	25. "Take the paper in your right hand." 26. "Fold it in half." 27. "Put it on the floor."	Understanding Complex Tasks
8. Show the person a written command and instruct the person to follow it.	28. "Close your eyes."	Reading Complex Tasks
9. Give the person a blank sheet of paper and pen and instruct the person to write.	29. "Write a complete sentence, whatever you want to write."	Writing
10. Give the person a blank sheet of paper and pen and show the person a picture of a complex design (interlocking pentagons). Instruct the person to copy the figure.	30. "Copy this drawing."	Visual spatial

Scoring

(Adapted from Mini-Mental State from Modified Cognitive Functioning Quiz. Folstein, Tolstein, McHugh, 1975.)

25 or higher: You're OK
24–21: Try it again.
20–10: Start doing those crossword puzzles.
9–0: You may want to have the person tested by a doctor.

Notes

We are grateful to the following who have given permission to use their materials.

Kirk, Thomas. "Diagnosis of Alzheimer's Disease Pushes Families to the Limit." New York, NY, November 5, 1998.

Pauluk, Mary. St. John Lutheran Home, Springfield, Minnesota.

Wiland-Bell. Reprinted from *And Thou Shalt Honor*. Rodale, Inc., Emmaus, PA: Rodale, Inc., 2002.

The drawings of the brain in Part V and Appendix 1 are adapted with permission from the chapter by Roger A. Brumback in *Ethical Foundations of Palliative Care for Alzheimer's Disease* by Ruth B. Purtilo and A.M.J. ten Have (eds). Baltimore: Johns Hopkins University Press, 2004.

COMMENTS AND SUGGESTIONS
PLEASE HELP US IMPROVE THIS HANDBOOK

Thank you for showing interest in *Alzheimer's Disease, The Dignity Within: A Handbook for Caregivers, Family, and Friends*. Your feedback will be helpful to future editions. We invite you to take a few minutes and answer the following questions:

How did you hear about this book?

_____

_____

_____

Where did you purchase/obtain your copy of the book?

_____

_____

_____

On a scale of 1 (being the weakest) to 5 (being the strongest), please rate what you found to be of most interest/helpful/enlightening.

Part 1: Being a Caregiver: Challenges and Solutions (1–2–3–4–5)
Because:

_____

_____

_____

_____

Part 2: The Reluctant Caregiver: A Husband and Wife's Personal Story (1–2–3–4–5)
Because:

_____

_____

_____

_____

Part 3: True Stories: Relationships between Persons Affected by the Disease Their Caregivers, Family Members, and Friends (1–2–3–4–5)
Because:

_____

_____

_____

_____

Part 4: Caregiving Styles: Three Ways to Respond (1–2–3–4–5)
Because:

_____

_____

_____

_____

Part 5: Alzheimer's Disease: Changes in the Brain (1–2–3–4–5)
Because:

_____

_____

_____

_____

Other:

_____

_____

Because:

_____

_____

_____

_____

Please identify yourself by completing the information below (Check all that apply.)

1. I am
   —— caregiver
   —— family member
   —— friend
   —— medical professional
   —— volunteer
   —— nursing home worker
   —— person diagnosed with Alzheimer's disease
   —— other

2. I am between the ages of
   —— 20–30
   —— 30–40
   —— 40–50
   —— 50–60
   —— 60–70
   —— 70–80
   —— 80–90

3. Name (Optional):

_____

4. E-mail:

_____

Please return your comments to:

CaringConcepts, Inc.
920 Branding Iron Drive
Elkhorn, NE 68022

Fax your responses to: (402) 289–0749

Thank you.

Index

J

K

L

M